STEP-BY-STEP

TAI
CHI

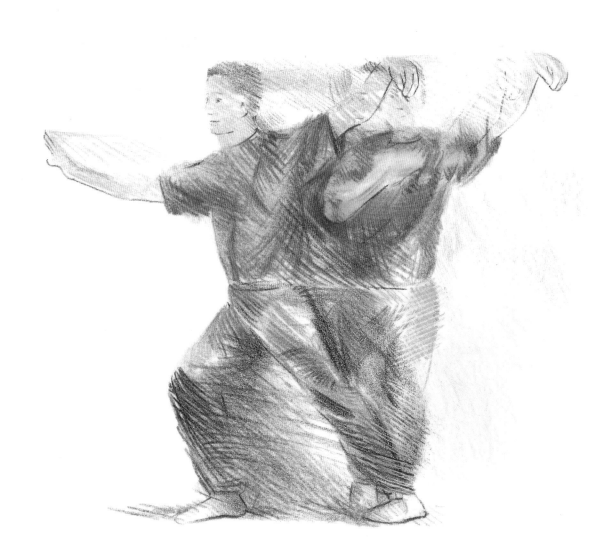

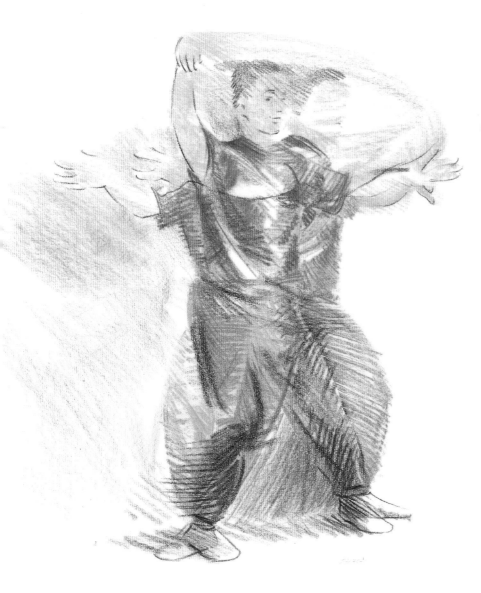

STEP-BY-STEP

TAI CHI

Master Lam Kam Chuen

A GAIA ORIGINAL

A FIRESIDE BOOK
Published by SIMON & SCHUSTER INC.

FIRESIDE
Rockefeller Center
1230 Avenue of the Americas
New York, New York 10020

First published in the United Kingdom in 1994 by
Gaia Books Ltd, 66 Charlotte Street, London W1P 1LR

Editorial	Pip Morgan
	Jonathan Hilton
Design	Sara Mathews
Illustration	Gordon Munro
Calligraphy	Master Lam Kam Chuen
Jacket Photography	Alex Wilson
Direction	Joss Pearson
	Patrick Nugent

Library of Congress Cataloging in Publication Data

Chuen, Lam Kam.
    Step-by-step tai chi / by Master Lam Kam Chuen.
        p.   cm.
    "A Gaia original".
    "A Fireside book".

    1. T'ai chi ch'uan.   I. Title.
GV504.C512 1994
613.7'148--dc20   94-7581
                                                               CIP

ISBN-13:   978-0-671-89247-0
ISBN-10:   0-671-89247-9
Printed and bound by Toppan in China
20 19 18 17 16 15 14 13

Author's acknowledgments

I hope that this book will help people in all walks of life and at all stages of growth to sustain and improve their health. I am sure that those who wish either to study Tai Chi or to broaden their grasp of it will find many treasures here. Many masters of Tai Chi, Chi Kung, and of the Chinese martial arts and medicine have made it possible for me to develop my own understanding of Tai Chi. Without Master Lung Tse Chung, from whom I first learned in Hong Kong, I would never have stepped into the world of Tai Chi. It was Professor Yu Yong Nian in Beijing who later showed me the heart of Zhan Zhuang Chi Kung, which I have incorporated in Lam style Tai Chi. What I have tried to do in this book is to present the fundamentals of what I have learned in a way that can be used in the West. I also owe an immense debt of gratitude to my wife Villisa, and to my three sons, Tin Yun, Tin Yu, and Tin Hun for their constant support and inspiration.

This book evolved as a result of my contact with countless students over the years. Those who volunteered to assist in the production of this book include William Bithell, Jill Chisholm, Maggie Coster, Richard Donkin, Pat Fitton, Pauline Harding, Beryl Heed, Lynn Jackson, Sue May, Howard Richmond, Steve Scarlett, Sean Stiles, Jill Sugden, Sarah Vicary, and Jean Willson. Particular thanks are due to Jane Ward for her thoughtful work in helping me elaborate and test the exercise routines throughout the book.

Richard Reoch devoted himself to preparing the English text on the basis of countless hours of oral instruction. As a result of his painstaking efforts, we hope that beginners will find our book straightforward and down-to-earth and that those who are already familiar with Tai Chi will discover from it the profound tradition of authentic Tai Chi.

I would also like to thank everyone at Gaia Books who made this book possible: Joss Pearson for persistently seeking international publishers; Eleanor Lines for her early advice on the text; Sara Mathews for developing the overall design, seeing through all the reference photography, and enthusiastically bringing each page to life; Gordon Munro for his meticulous drawings; Jonathan Hilton for his editing of the manuscript; and Pip Morgan for his wise editorial guidance.

CONTENTS

ABOUT THE AUTHOR

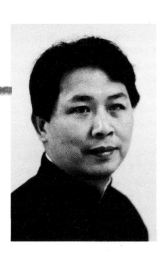

Master Lam Kam Chuen is a recognized master of the arts of Tai Chi and Chi Kung, and a practitioner of traditional Chinese medicine. He was born in Hong Kong shortly after World War II and at a very early age began training in Chinese martial arts.

Studying under masters such as Lung Tse Chung and Yim Sheung Mo (both of whom were disciples of Ku Yue Chang, known throughout China as "The King of Iron Palm"), he was trained in Choy Lee Fut, Northern Shaolin Kung Fu and Iron Palm, as well as Tai Chi.

He then studied Chinese medicine, becoming a qualified bonesetter and herbalist, and opened a school and clinic in Hong Kong. He also undertook the study of Chi Kung, a system for the cultivation of internal energy in the body. Using his medical skills and his knowledge of Chi Kung he began to develop a new form of Tai Chi, now known as Lam Style Tai Chi.

Master Lam came to the West in 1976 when he became the first Tai Chi instructor appointed to teach in the Inner London Education Authority. In 1987 he gave the first European demonstration of the art of Zhan Zhuang Chi Kung, which he studied in Beijing under Professor Yu Yong Nian, the world's leading authority. He now teaches and practices medicine at The Lam Clinic in London's Chinatown.

Following the widely acclaimed BBC series, "The Way of the Warrior", Master Lam was invited to act as consultant to the sequel publication, *The Way of Harmony*. This was followed by his ground-breaking work published by Gaia Books, *The Way of Energy*, introducing the Zhan Zhuang system of "Standing Like a Tree".

A LIFETIME'S STUDY

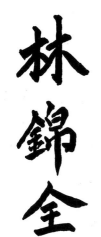

"When I was 12 years old I was sent to a master of the martial arts in Hong Kong. He wanted me to learn Tai Chi, but I was much keener on the hard kicks and punches of Southern and Northern Shaolin Kung Fu. In fact, I was a very unwilling student of Tai Chi!

One day when I was practicing Kung Fu, I completely seized up. My master ordered me to do my Tai Chi exercises. Even though the movements were soft and gentle, my body began to sweat profusely. Next day I had completely recovered. I pondered the powerful effect that the gentle Tai Chi had produced in me – it was the beginning of a lifetime's study.

When my master died a few years later I sought out teachers in Hong Kong, in China, and in Taiwan. Finally I was accepted as a student by an old monk who revealed a great deal to me. Together with what he taught me and my studies of Chinese medicine, I began to understand the inner workings of this healing system.

It was at that stage that I discovered the Zhan Zhuang system of Chi Kung. Literally meaning 'Standing like a Tree', this method of developing the Chi – vital energy – was remarkable. I began to work on ways to integrate it into my Tai Chi.

For 10 years I worked at developing a system that would merge the benefits of everything I had learned. Originally I used it just for myself. When I came to the West, I realized that it could be adapted and taught to others. That is the basis of this book."

INTRODUCTION

MOVING HARMONY

Thousands of people are looking for some way to stay fit and healthy. They don't want to sign up for gymnastics, nor do they want to spend hours jogging or lifting weights. They don't want to end up sweating, breathless, and in pain. This book is the answer to their plea.

Tai Chi has evolved through the ages as a highly refined system of exercise and personal development. It is absorbing, but it is not exhausting or stressful. It consists of a series of slow, continuous movements designed to relax and develop the whole body. One of its great attractions is that, no matter what your age, you can practice its full range of movements.

The aim of the carefully structured sequence of movements is to build up the body's internal strength, suppleness, and stamina. The unique quality of this ancient art is being used increasingly for its health-giving properties. Once learned, it is a treasure that will last you a lifetime.

Getting started

One of the appealing things about Tai Chi is that you don't need anything special to be able to learn it. You do not need special clothing or equipment; you do not need to go somewhere special to do it; you do not need to learn Chinese or believe in any religion; you do not have to reorganize your life or stick to a rigid new exercise schedule. And no matter how little you do or how slow your progress, you can be certain in your own mind that with the help of this book the instructions you are following are authentic, accurate, and perfectly safe.

It is best to try doing a little Tai Chi every day. This will help to keep your memory fresh and produce the best results, particularly if you are interested in Tai Chi for stress relief. Normally, it is best to practice Tai Chi first thing in the morning. If this is not possible, then just try to fit it in whenever you can. You can wear almost anything you like, but loose, comfortable clothes are best. You can wear soft, flat shoes or socks. Tai Chi is traditionally practiced in the open air. If you do it indoors; try to use an airy, well-ventilated room. You do not need much space for Tai Chi. You can do almost everything in this book in an area large enough for you to be able to swing your arms around freely .

Stress release

Tai Chi is a proven antidote to stress. The stress reaction in the human body involves the "fight or flight" syndrome. This is the reaction of your nervous system to events that cause you to feel under pressure. Your bodily functions go on a sort of "war footing": blood pressure rises; blood is drained from the stomach, intestines, skin, and extremities; the heart speeds up; the respiratory rate increases and the brain readies itself for conflict.

Many of the pressures of daily life mean that our whole biological system is on this sort of constant alert, even in sleep. We see the results around us everywhere: hypertension, migraines, asthma, all manner of aches and pains, some menstrual difficulties, depression, and heart attacks.

Some people find release through sports and aerobic exercise. These help to disperse tension and strengthen the respiratory, muscular, and cardiovascular systems. But the benefits are often offset by the effects of competition or the punishment we put our bodies through.

Other people try to relax by "getting away from it all". The most extreme form of this is secluded meditation. The effects are well known: a slower pulse and respiratory rate, improved digestion, greater mental alertness, and tranquillity. The brain operates at a different register, one more akin to the depths of the sea than to the turbulent waves to be found on the surface. But many people find that this state of tranquillity is extremely difficult to preserve once they return to the rest of their lives and the world in which they daily operate.

The beauty of Tai Chi is that it offers a middle course between these extremes — and it includes the benefits of both. It achieves this without involving either the punishment of violent exercise or the shock of re-entry to the world after meditative withdrawal.

The health benefits

We all tend to store up the effects of stress in our musculature, as everybody with a pain in the neck or a stiff or frozen shoulder knows full well. Bodybuilding or vigorous sports activities strengthen certain muscles, but do not train the muscles to tolerate pressure without tension. Indeed, the build up of lactic acid leads to muscular fatigue, as every athlete can tell you!

Tai Chi is different, however. It brings many muscles into play, but it does so in a way that enables both balanced development and relaxation. Slow movements require endurance rather than force, and so they develop a different type of muscle fiber. The result is that our muscular response to stress changes over time and we become progressively relieved of the burden of accumulated physical tension.

The changes in our muscles also start to improve our posture. The back muscles learn to relax, enabling them to elongate. The ligaments become more supple and so the movement of the entire spinal column tends to be freer and more comfortable.

Stiffness of the joints is often related to stress. The tension in our muscles impedes the smooth movement of our joints, and so they start to degenerate. Tai Chi addresses this problem by working on the elasticity and strength of all the major joints. The sustained rotations and flowing movements encourage the health of the cartilaginous surfaces on the bone ends. In this way, the exercises help to retard degeneration of the joints and act as an anti-stress massage.

Recently, scientists have been studying the internal physiological benefits of Tai Chi. One index they use to measure the effects is cardiorespiratory fitness – the maximum amount of oxygen a person is capable of using. Measurements comparing Tai Chi practitioners and others have shown that if you practice Tai Chi regularly, your cardiorespiratory fitness improves, particularly if you were out of condition in the first place.

Tai Chi and the mind

Just as Tai Chi improves the health of the body, it also has a profound effect on the nervous system. Those who regularly practice Tai Chi attest to their improved powers of concentration, coordination, and inner balance. It has often been described as a form of "moving meditation", and studies of the brain waves of Tai Chi practitioners confirm the accuracy of this description.

Tai Chi, therefore, not only facilitates a state of wakeful relaxation, but its effects are also at the heart of health and regeneration. The Chinese have known of Tai Chi's healing power for centuries, employing it to combat a wide range of disorders including heart and circulation problems, addictions, arthritic conditions, muscle injuries, asthma, and nervous disturbances.

An ancient heritage

For ages, the art of Tai Chi was a secret heritage of just a small number of families living in China. Almost exclusively, parents passed the knowledge on to their children. Only in the 20th century has Tai Chi been taught and practiced so widely. Five styles have become the best known. Each is named after the master who developed it: Chen, Yang, Wu, Shin, and Ng. Each has its own exercises and sequences of continuous movements known as a "form". The sequence that you will be introduced to in Part Two of this book, the Small Circle Form, includes some of the most important movements common to all the classical Tai Chi styles.

Tai Chi: its meaning

The full name in Chinese is Tai Chi Chuan. The correct English pronunciation is normally Tie (as in bow tie) Chee (as in cheetah) Chwan (the "a" is long, as in want). There are many literal translations given for these three words. Often the translation is "supreme ultimate fist". Some people simply say "shadow boxing".

I tell my students that the most important thing in translation is to convey the real meaning that lies behind the characters. To do that, I point to the Tai Chi symbol: the two semicircles of light and dark that make a complete circle as they constantly merge into each other. Many people know this as the symbol of Yin and Yang. In fact, the symbol is literally called "the Tai Chi" in Chinese. So this is the real spirit of Tai Chi Chuan. I call it "moving harmony".

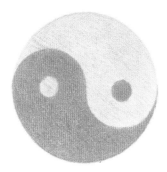

太極拳基礎

PART **1**

TAI CHI FOUNDATIONS

Tai Chi works on your body and your mind at the same time. The movements not only relax your muscles, they calm your nerves as well. If you are using this book to teach yourself Tai Chi, it is important to understand that the very first lesson of Tai Chi is to relax.

All the movements are done slowly and gently. To give you an idea of the timing, experiment with Exercise Seven on page 26, Playing the Accordion. Time yourself as you move an imaginary accordion between your hands, calmly breathing in and out with the movements. Three complete in and out movements can take you about half a minute. At first you may find that just too difficult, making you tense. So you will need to adjust to find your own comfortable, but calm, pace. But unlike other exercise systems where you work hard at speeding up as you get better, in Tai Chi, as we slow down we improve !

The interplay of stillness and movement is fundamental to Tai Chi, as it is to life. You will find that each exercise begins and ends with standing still for a few seconds. This is not an empty pause in between the exercises. It is part of the exercise. Please don't skip ahead if you are feeling fine or are in a rush. The stillness is essential. It is not empty. Without it, your movements will be without energy. Both the stillness and the movement are your Tai Chi.

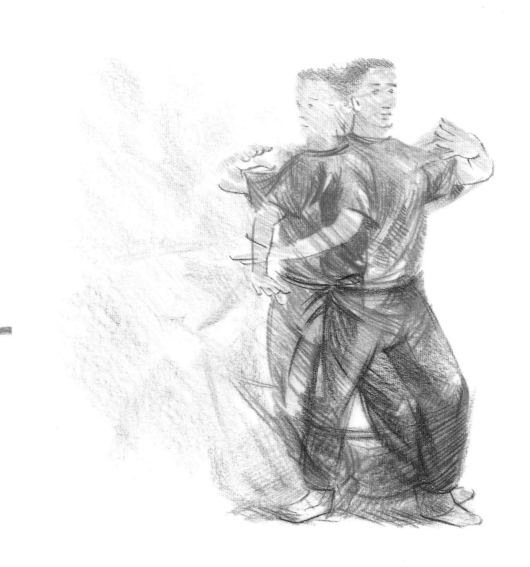

CHAPTER ONE

FUNDAMENTAL MOVEMENTS

This set of basic exercises is designed to relax and tone all the major joints in your body. Starting with the neck, you work down through your entire frame. For the best results from these exercises, you should work through the full set in the correct order.

The movements are simple to learn. Most of them are based on the natural action of the joints when they are relaxed and free from tension. For this reason, if you are just starting to learn Tai Chi you should begin with this sequence to ensure that you develop a good foundation of smooth, relaxed movement.

These fundamental exercises are presented in a way that will be particularly helpful to anyone who has never done slow exercise before. They are ideal if you are out of shape, recuperating from an illness or a physical injury, or are elderly. Follow the instructions carefully, go slowly, and don't strain yourself in any movement and the benefits can be remarkable.

The exercises are based on two principles. First, there is a great deal of tension in our joints and their associated muscles. It is essential, therefore, to learn how to relax these areas in order to keep them supple and to help overcome the damaging effects tension has on the body. Second, all our major energy pathways pass through the joints. If tension exists there, then the natural flow of energy in the body will be blocked, leading to increased stress and, eventually, illness. So these exercises, simple as they may seem at first, meet some of our most fundamental needs.

Each exercise is described in detail, including the starting position for each, the precise movement, the pauses, and the all-important concluding moments of stillness. Many of these features are common to each exercise, but they are repeated so that you can be sure that at each stage you know exactly what you are supposed to be doing.

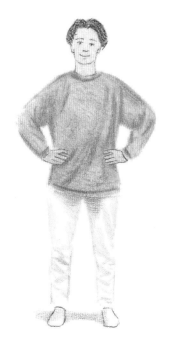 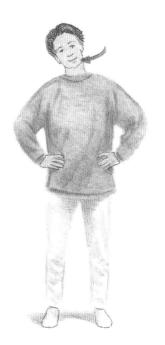 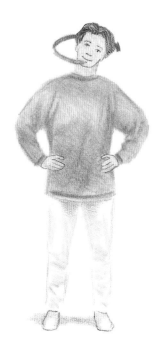

EXERCISE 1   RELAXING THE NECK

1 Stand with your feet shoulder-width apart, facing forward. Rest your hands on your hips. Relax your shoulders and let your elbows sink gently down. Breathe calmly and naturally.

2 Keep your body still. Imagine that your head is floating on top of your body like a globe. Gently start to let your head roll around in a clockwise direction (your head moves first toward the right). This movement should be smooth and effortless. The idea is just to release the tension in your neck, not to stretch it.

3 Keeping your eyes open, make three gentle circles. After the third circle, pause with your head facing straight ahead. Stay like that for one second.

Now make three gentle circles with your head moving counter-clockwise. Again, finish with your head facing forward. Lower both hands slowly down to your sides. Stand still for a second or two before going on to the next exercise.

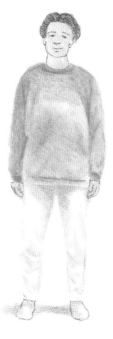
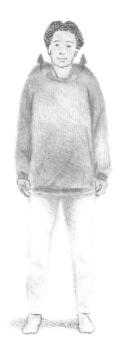
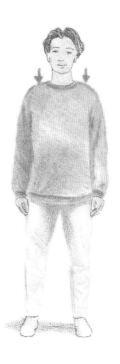

EXERCISE 2 LOWERING THE SHOULDERS

1 Stand in the same relaxed position as in the previous exercise. Keep your feet facing forward, shoulder-width apart. Leave your hands hanging loosely and comfortably down by your sides.

2 Breathe in and slowly raise both shoulders. Do this without tensing or moving the rest of your body.

3 Breathe out and gently lower both shoulders. Let your hands hang loosely down at your sides as you do this. When your hands have dropped down as far as they can go, leave them in that position for one second. Repeat the raising and lowering movement of your shoulders six times at a rate that is comfortable for you, without forcing either your breathing or movements. Stand still for a second or two to relax further when you have finished.

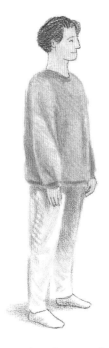
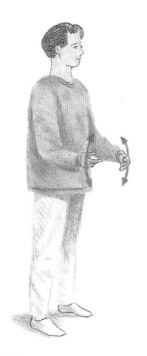
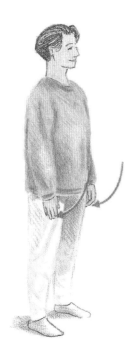

EXERCISE 3   SHAKING THE HANDS

1 Stand in the relaxed position. Keep your feet facing forward, shoulder–width apart. Raise your hands gently up in front of your belly, as if lifting a large balloon.

2 Begin to shake your hands as if you were shaking water off them. Continuously shake your hands while you complete three full, smooth breaths. Keep your hands in front of your belly. Be sure that your shoulders and neck are relaxed throughout.

3 Then lower your hands to your sides and stand still for a second or two before going on to the next exercise.

2◆ *Shake your hands loosely from the wrists with your fingers completely relaxed.*

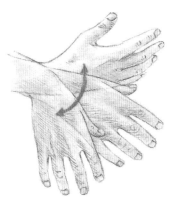

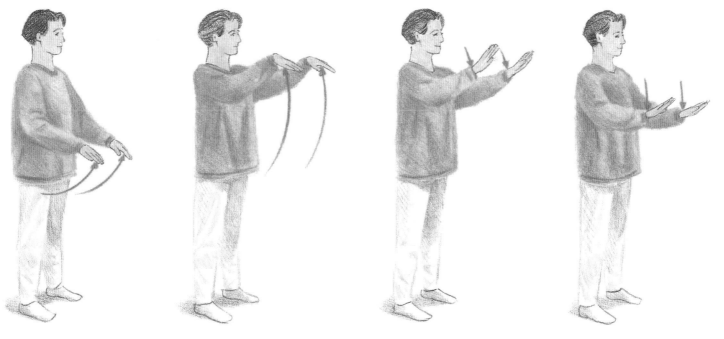

EXERCISE 4 PAINTING THE WALL

1 Stay in the relaxed standing position with your feet facing forward, shoulder-width apart. Imagine that your hands are paint brushes that are held by your wrists and that your fingers are the bristles of the brushes. Start to raise your hands.

2 Raise your hands gently up as if you were painting a wall in front of you with long vertical strokes. Your hands move smoothly, like brushes. Keep your shoulders relaxed as your arms move. As you brush up, breathe in gently.

3 The upward stroke is complete when your hands are at head height. Then start to lower your wrists so that your hands, like paint brushes, are tilted upward ready to begin brushing back down.

4 Brush back down the wall, finishing at about waist level. As your arms come down, breathe out. Your fingers and wrists should be as flexible as possible. Complete six raising and lowering movements of the arms. Then stand still for a second or two at the end of the exercise.

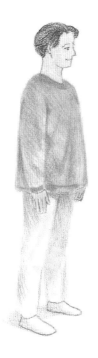
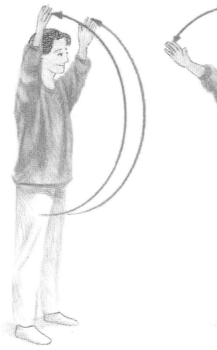
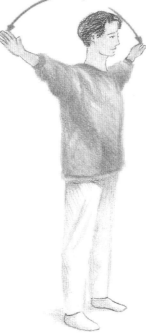
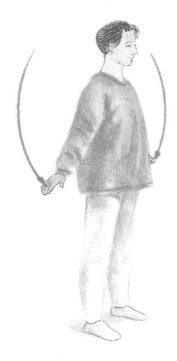

EXERCISE 5 TWO FULL MOONS

1 Stay in the relaxed standing position, feet facing forward, shoulder-width apart. Let your hands hang loosely down at your sides.

2 Slowly raise both arms in front of you, allowing a little relaxation in the elbows and wrists. As your arms come up, breathe in. Continue the motion of the arms up and around, making large circles like two full moons. Keep your shoulders relaxed and do not hunch them up as you move your arms.

3 As your arms circle back down, breathe out. Adjust the speed of your arm movements to fit comfortably with your natural breathing.

4 At the end of the circle, your arms come down beside you in preparation for the start of the next circle. Look to the front and keep the rest of your body steady. Make six full circles. Lower your hands by your sides 28 at the end and pause for a second or two before going on to the next exercise.

EXERCISE 6   BRUSHING THE AIR

1 Stay in the relaxed standing position, feet facing forward, shoulder-width apart. This will be the reverse movement of the previous exercise.

2 Slowly bring your arms up and out behind you. As your arms come up behind you, breathe in. Keep your shoulders relaxed and do not hunch them up as you move your arms.

3 Continue the slow movement of both of your arms, up past your head.

4 As your hands come forward, breathe out. Imagine that you are brushing the air in front of you with your fingers. Continue the smooth circular movement of your arms without stopping. Relax your hands. Adjust the speed of your arm movements to fit comfortably with your natural breathing. Look to the front and keep the rest of your body steady. Make six full circles. Rest your arms by your sides for a second or two when you have finished the circles.

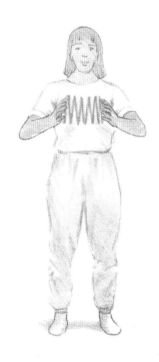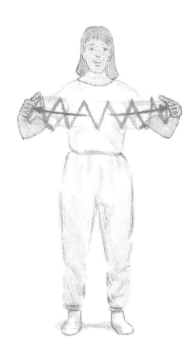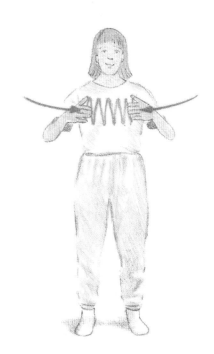

EXERCISE 7   PLAYING THE ACCORDION

1 Stand in the relaxed position with your feet facing forward, shoulder-width apart. Raise your hands gently up in front of your chest as if you were about to start playing the accordion.

2 Move your arms gently outward as if you were opening the bellows of the accordion. Breathe in as you do this.

3 Bring your arms gently back in as if you were closing the bellows. Breathe out as you do this. Make six full movements, matching your breathing to the movement of the accordion. Keep your shoulders and neck relaxed throughout and let your wrists be as flexible as possible. Gently lower your hands to your sides at the end and pause for a second or two.

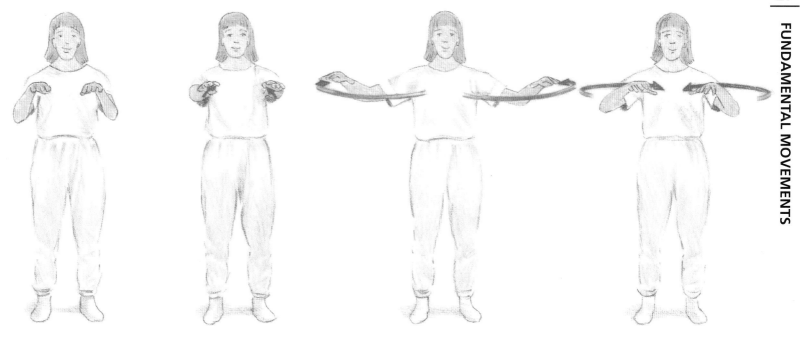

EXERCISE 8 SWIMMING ON LAND

1 Continue standing in the relaxed position, feet facing the front, shoulder-width apart. Raise your hands gently up to chest height as if you were about to begin to swim using the breast stroke. Breathe in.

2 Extend your arms forward as if you were moving ahead in the water. Keep your movement very smooth and calm. As your arms move forward, breathe out. Keep looking forward with your head up.

3 As in the breast stroke, your arms move apart from each other after they extend forward.

4 Complete the breast stroke movement by bringing both hands back toward your chest in gentle circles. Breathe in as your hands come back to your chest. Make six complete strokes. Gently lower your arms and stay still for a second or two.

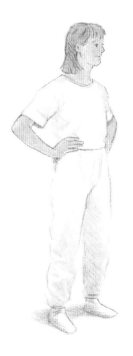
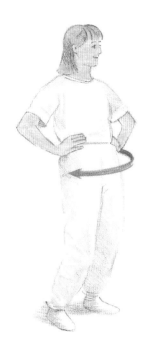
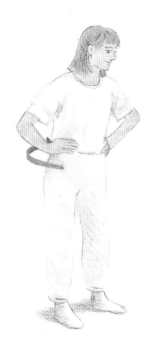
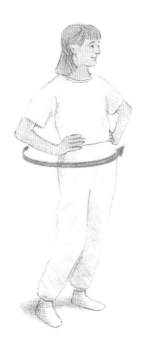

EXERCISE 9   HIP CIRCLES

1 Stay in the relaxed position, with your feet facing forward, shoulder-width apart. Rest your hands on your hips. Let your shoulders and elbows drop gently down.

2 Slowly move your hips in a large circle, starting in a clockwise direction (your hips move first toward the right).

3 As you make the full circle with your hips, imagine your head is suspended by a fine thread and it is only your hips that circle around. Your knees should be straight and steady. Breathe calmly and naturally. Make three large circles.

4 Then make large hip circles in the opposite direction, moving counter-clockwise. Keep your head up and your knees straight. Make three large circles, breathing naturally all the time. Then come to rest, standing still for a second or two.

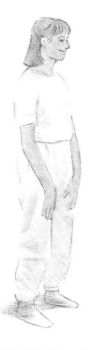 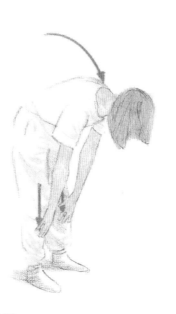 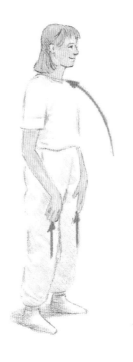

EXERCISE 10 BENDING FORWARD

1 Stand in the relaxed position, feet facing forward, shoulder-width apart. Relax your hands. Spread your fingers slightly apart and gently place your hands on the front of your thighs. Your fingers should be pointing toward your feet.

2 Slowly bend forward from the waist, your back forming a natural curve. Let your hands slide lightly down your thighs. Always keep the hands touching your legs so that you can brace yourself if you lose balance. Gradually go down as far as you can without bending your knees. As you go down, breathe out. Try to touch your toes, but don't force the movement. Wherever you stop, hold the position for one second.

3 Slowly come up, sliding your hands up your legs. This will ensure the correct position of your spine. Breathe in as you come up. Stay still for one second. Make three of these forward bends. Then stand fully up and return your hands to your sides. Pause at the end for a second or two before going on to the next exercise.

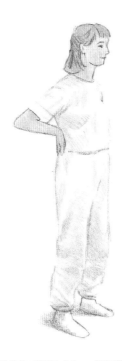
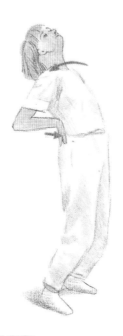
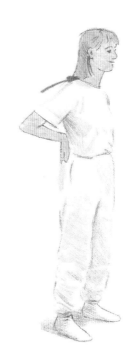

EXERCISE 11   BENDING BACKWARD

1 Remain in the relaxed standing position, your feet facing forward, shoulder-width apart. Relax your hands. Spread your fingers slightly apart and rest your hands against the small of your back. Your fingers should be angled naturally toward your buttocks.

2 Slowly bend backward from the waist, using your hands to push your waist forward for balance. As you go back, allow your knees to bend slightly. This causes your weight to come gradually forward on to the balls of your feet, but both heels should remain in contact with the floor. Look slightly upward. As you bend back, breathe out. Hold the position for one second.

3 Slowly come back up to the upright position, breathing in as you do. Stay still for one second. Make three of these bends, going back each time only as far as you comfortably can. Don't overdo the stretch. Come back to a natural vertical position, bring your hands back to your sides, and stand still for a second or two.

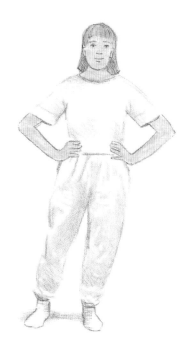 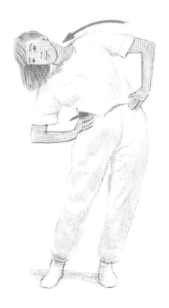 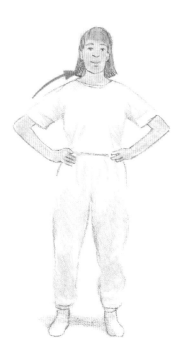

EXERCISE 12   BENDING TO THE SIDE

1 Continue in the relaxed position, feet facing forward, shoulder-width apart. Rest your hands on your hips. Let your shoulders and elbows drop gently down. Shift your weight on to your left foot, keeping both legs straight.

2 Press your right hand into your hip as you lower your body over to the right side. Let your head gently follow the movement. Bend to the side as far as you are able, keeping the soles of both feet on the ground. Breathe out as you bend. Hold the position for one second.

3 Slowly straighten up, breathing in. When you come up transfer your weight back from the left foot so that it is evenly centered over both feet. Stay still for one second. Repeat the whole movement, bending to the right three times. Then shift your weight to the right foot and make three bends to the left side. Don't forget to center your weight over both feet after each bend. At the end, return to the upright, centered position and pause for a second or two, keeping your hands on your hips.

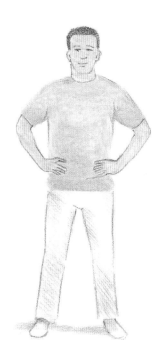
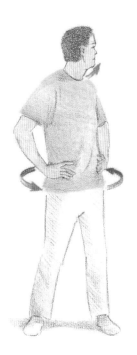
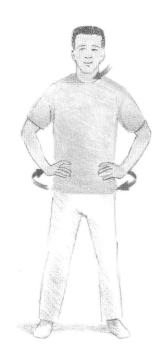

EXERCISE 13 LOOKING BACK AT THE MOON

1 Stand with your weight centered over both feet. Face forward. Rest your hands on your hips. Let your shoulders and elbows drop gently down.

2 Very slowly turn your whole upper body and waist around to the left, keeping your feet firmly in position. When you have turned around as far as you can, continue the movement by slightly lifting your head and looking up a little, as if gazing back at the moon over your shoulder. Breathe out as you turn. Hold the position for one second.

3 Very slowly turn back toward the front. Breathe in as you do this. Stay facing the front for one second. Repeat the turn to the other side. Make six turns altogether, alternately turning to the left and right. Don't forget to synchronize your breathing with the movement and to pause for one second at the end of each turn. At the end, return to face the front, lower your hands to your sides, and stand still for a second or two.

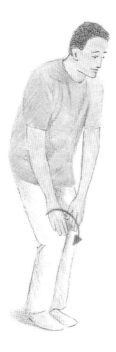
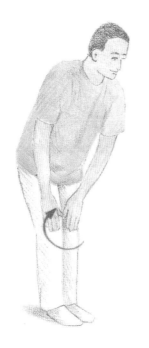
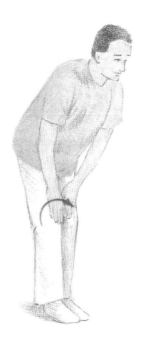
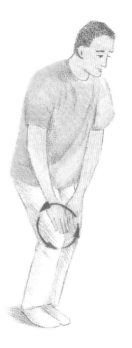

EXERCISE 14 KNEE CIRCLES

1 Put your feet together. Bend your knees slightly and lower your hands so that you can just touch your knees with your fingertips. Look at a point on the floor about 6 feet (2m) in front of you, in order to achieve the correct position for your neck and head.

2 Keeping your fingertips resting on your knees and with your knees together, make smooth circles with your knees starting in a clockwise direction (your knees start to circle first toward the right).

3 Try to keep the soles of your feet flat on the floor as your knees move in circles. Avoid tensing your neck and back. Breathe naturally. Make six gentle clockwise circles.

4 When you have completed the clockwise circles, reverse direction and make six counter-clockwise circles. Your feet may tend to wiggle around on the floor; try to keep them flat. Then slowly come back up to the relaxed standing position and stay still until your breathing and heart rate are normal.

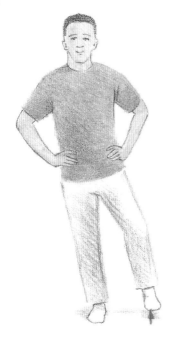

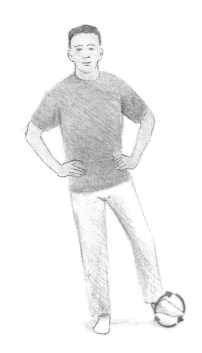

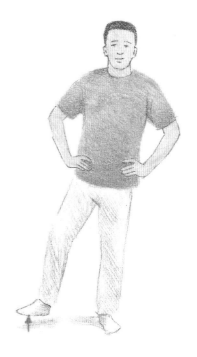

EXERCISE 15   ANKLE CIRCLES

1 Remain in the standing position and put your hands on your hips. Shift your weight over to your right foot and lift your left foot about 6 inches (15cm) off the ground.

2 Make three small circles with your left ankle, moving your foot in a counter-clockwise direction (the toes move first toward the left). Breathe naturally. Then lower your left foot, center your weight, and pause for one second.

2♦ *Each of the ankle circles begins with the foot moving to the side away from the body. This detail shows the right foot.*

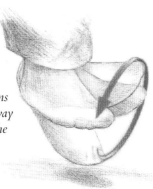

3 Then shift your weight over to your left foot and lift your right foot off the ground. Make three small circles with your right ankle in a clockwise direction (the toes move first toward the right). Breathe naturally. Then lower your right foot, center your weight over both feet, and stand still for one or two seconds.

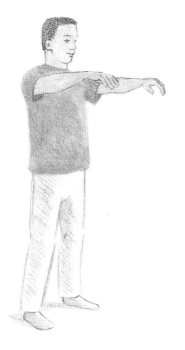
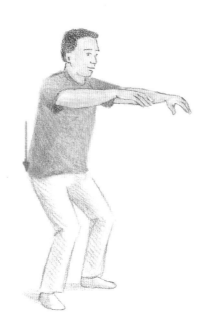
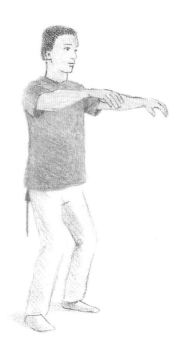

EXERCISE 16 **SITTING DOWN**

1 Stand in the relaxed position, with your feet facing forward, shoulder-width apart. Slowly raise your arms up in front of you to chest height. As you do this, breathe in.

2 Slowly lower your buttocks as if you were going to sit down in a chair. Your extended arms will help keep you balanced. Keep both feet firmly on the floor. Breathe out as you go down. Sink as far down as you can. When you have gone down as far as you can, hold the position for one second.

3 Slowly stand up, breathing in as you move. When you are fully upright, stay still for one second. Then repeat the entire movement three times. When you stand up for the last time, lower your arms and rest for a second or two.

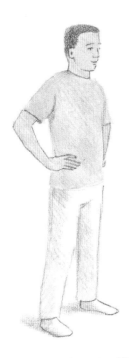
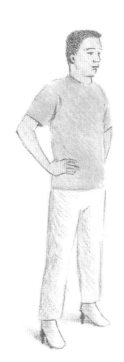
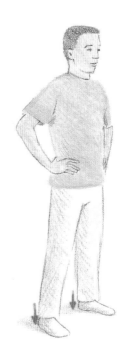

EXERCISE 17 RISING ON YOUR TOES

1 Begin in the standing position, feet facing forward, shoulder-width apart. Rest your hands on your hips. Breathe in to start.

2 Rise up on your toes as you breathe out. Keep your neck and shoulders completely relaxed. Keep your balance without leaning backward. When you are up on your toes, hold the position until you have completely exhaled.

3 When you have completely exhaled, slowly lower yourself back down so that your feet are flat on the floor again. Breathe in as you do this. Complete the rising and lowering movement six times. Then rest your hands by your side and stay still for one or two seconds.

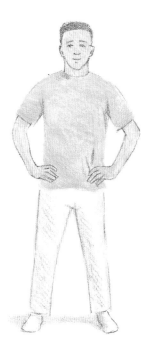 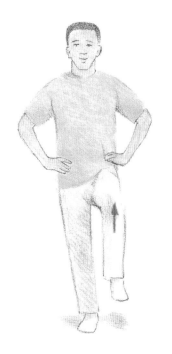 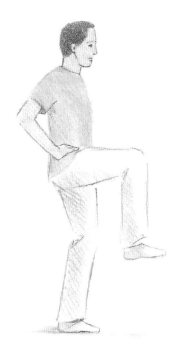

EXERCISE 18 LIFTING THE KNEES

1 Continue in the standing position with your feet facing forward, shoulder-width apart. Place your hands on your hips and look straight ahead.

2 Shift your weight on to your right foot. Gently lift your left foot until your knee is level with your hip (or only as far up as you can comfortably lift it off the floor), and gently lower it back down to the ground. Breathe naturally.

3 Now shift the weight over to the left foot. Gently lift and lower your right foot in the same way. As this side view shows, your head remains upright and your back straight. Complete six liftings and lowerings. Then stand still, lower your hands by your sides, and rest in that position for a moment so that the benefits of all these movements can flow in a balanced, relaxed way through your system.

EXERCISE ROUTINES

Working through the full set of 18 fundamental exercises gently and slowly, as described on the preceding pages, takes just under 10 minutes. You should start at this level, carefully making all the movements in order, pausing briefly in between each one, until you are familiar with the full set. The number of repetitions to start with for each exercise is set out in Level 1 on the chart opposite.

If you are unfamiliar with this type of slow exercise, or you are out of shape, in poor health, or elderly, take your time and do them as gently as possible. This way, without straining yourself, you will start to make progress each time you do them. Some people may prefer to remain at this basic level, doing the movements as best they can. Even if this is the only exercise you can take, it will be of great benefit to you.

Once you are familiar with the exercises, and if you find that you can do them fairly easily, there are two further levels set out on the chart opposite. So, for example, you proceed to making four gentle circles of the head at Level 2, then six circles at Level 3, and so on. Maintain the calm, steady pace throughout. It is essential for Tai Chi exercise that you keep to the discipline of doing all movements slowly and evenly.

Try to do these exercises every day. The continuous repetition will make all the difference to your health and it will progressively relax your body and mind.

EXERCISE ROUTINE	Level 1	Level 2	Level 3
	Number of repetitions		
Exercise 1 Relaxing the neck	3 each way	4 each way	6 each way
Exercise 2 Lowering the shoulders	6	6	6
Exercise 3 Shaking the hands	3 breaths	4 breaths	6 breaths
Exercise 4 Painting the wall	6	9	12
Exercise 5 Two full moons	6	9	12
Exercise 6 Brushing the air	6	9	12
Exercise 7 Playing the accordion	6	9	12
Exercise 8 Swimming on land	6	9	12
Exercise 9 Hip circles	3 each way	4 each way	6 each way
Exercise 10 Bending forward	3	4	6
Exercise 11 Bending backward	3	4	6
Exercise 12 Bending to the side	3 each side	4 each side	6 each side
Exercise 13 Looking back at the moon	3 each way	4 each way	6 each way
Exercise 14 Knee circles	6 each way	12 each way	30 each way
Exercise 15 Ankle circles	3 each foot	4 each foot	6 each foot
Exercise 16 Sitting down	3	6	12
Exercise 17 Rising on your toes	6	9	12
Exercise 18 Lifting the knees	3 each leg	6 each leg	12 each leg

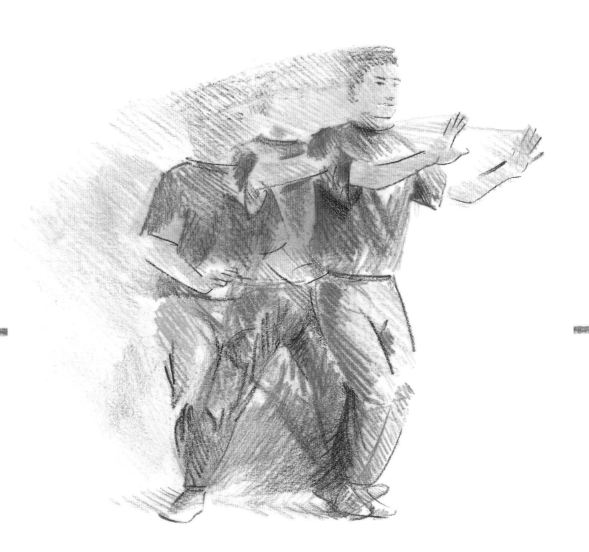

CHAPTER TWO

STRENGTH AND MOTION

These exercises are designed to develop inner strength and muscle control. Most of the movements are found in the sequence of 108 continuous movements of classical Tai Chi forms. They are presented as separate movements here so that you can utilize them as exercises for your own development. If you are already familiar with a Tai Chi form, then nothing in these exercises will in any way disturb the form you already know. They will, in fact, help you to grow into it.

If you are a complete beginner, you will find that practicing these exercises regularly will greatly aid your ability to learn in a Tai Chi class at some later stage. If you do not intend to learn a Tai Chi form (or have trouble doing so), practicing these movements will give you much of the benefit that other people derive from the repeated practice of a form. You can practice these 18 exercises as a full sequence or you can use them individually to help develop your body movement. The exercise routines at the end of the chapter will guide you in this.

In the exercises that follow in this chapter, you will need to stand with your knees bent – you will be reminded of this at the beginning of each exercise. Although only a simple differ-ence, it is a vitally important one. It is essential training to strengthen your legs, for example, and to develop your stamina and increase the flow of your internal energy. It also develops that sense of connection with the earth, a concept that we call being "rooted". In time, you will become firm on your feet – like a tree planted in the earth. As in Chapter One, each time you complete an exercise, stand relaxed and still for several seconds before moving on to the next one. This short period of calm is essential for the long-term development of your inner power and balance.

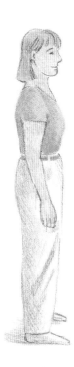 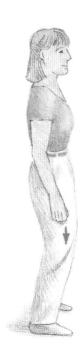

EXERCISE 19   STANDING IN THE WU CHI POSITION

This standing position exercise is known in Chinese as "Wu Chi" – the position of primal energy. You should practice it at the beginning of all your training from this point onward.

1 Stand with your feet facing forward, shoulder-width apart. Be certain that your toes are pointing directly ahead and not outward at an angle. Let your hands hang loosely by your sides and relax your shoulders. Your gaze should be straight ahead. Imagine that your head is lightly suspended from a fine thread.

2 Slowly bend both knees so that you lower yourself by about 2 inches (5cm). Be careful to ensure that your weight is evenly distributed over both feet and that it is centered in the middle of the soles of your feet. Check that your knees are not bent forward beyond your toes and that your upper body is still upright and relaxed. Stand calmly in this position, without moving, for two to three minutes. Breathe calmly and naturally.

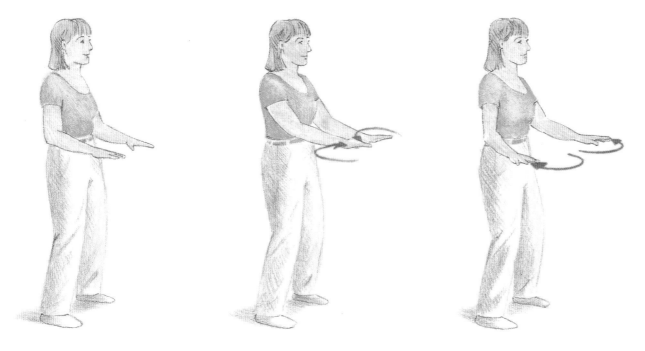

EXERCISE 20 POLISHING THE DESK

1 Stand in the Wu Chi position with your knees slightly bent. Lift your hands in front of your belly and turn them so that the palms face the floor and the fingers point toward the front.

2 Relax your hands and gently spread your fingers a little. Start making small, smooth circles opening outward with both hands, as if you were polishing the top of a desk.

3 Keep your hands flat and relaxed. Breathe naturally. Make 10 outward circles. Then, keeping your body still and with your hands still level with your belly, reverse the direction of the polishing and make another 10 circles with your hands. You may increase the number of circles up to 30 in each direction.

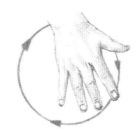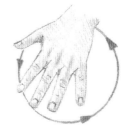

3◆ *With both hands make circles that move toward each other and then outward.*

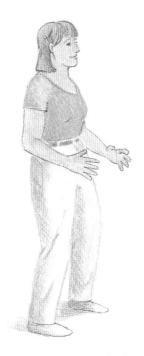 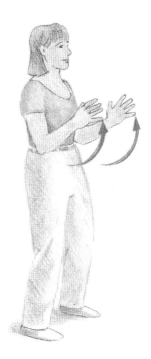 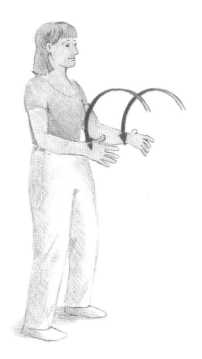

EXERCISE 21 **ROLLING THE BALLOON**

1 Stand in the Wu Chi position with your knees slightly bent and with your hands in front of your belly. Keep your hands relaxed and your fingers gently spread.

2 Imagine that you are holding a balloon between your palms. Start moving the balloon around in smooth circles that open outward from your belly, up to chest height and then back in and down toward your belly. Your elbows are loosely bent and move naturally with the movement of your arms. As you roll the balloon outward and upward, breathe out.

3 As the balloon comes down and in toward your belly, breathe in. Make between 10 and 30 of these circles.

Then, keeping your body still and with your hands still level with the belly, reverse the direction of the balloon. Always breathe out as your hands move outward and breathe in as your hands come in toward your body. Make a minimum of 10 circles and up to 30 circles for greater benefit.

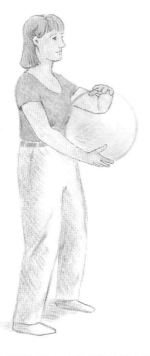
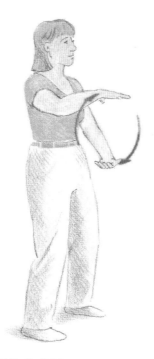
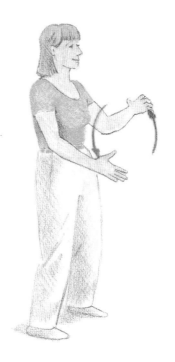

EXERCISE 22   TURNING THE BALLOON

1 Stand in the Wu Chi position with your knees slightly bent. Hold your left hand so that it is a comfortable distance in front of you, opposite your chest, palm facing downward. Your right hand should be level with your navel, the palm facing upward. It is as if you were holding a balloon between your two hands. Your fingers should be gently spread.

2 Turn the imaginary balloon over so that your right hand comes on top and your left hand ends up underneath. Make sure that there is a lot of space under your armpit as you make this movement, and that the joints from your shoulders to your wrists and fingers are all relaxed as you move.

3 Then turn the balloon back over the other way, so that your left hand comes back up on top and your right hand goes underneath. There is no special breathing for this exercise: just breathe naturally. Make a minimum of 10 turnings of the balloon and up to 30 to really loosen up the joints.

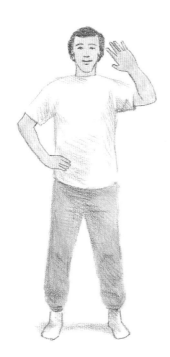
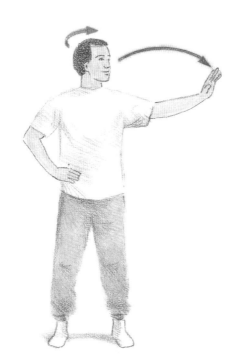
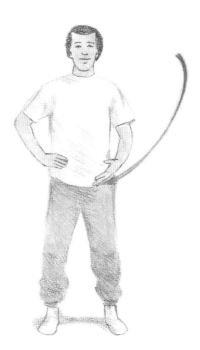

EXERCISE 23   OPENING THE CURTAIN

1 Stand in the Wu Chi position with your knees slightly bent. Place your right hand on your hip. Hold your left hand up beside your head, the palm turned to face outward, with the fingers gently spread.

2 Move your left hand over to the left as if you were opening a curtain. Move your hand nearly as far as you can, but without straightening either the elbow or wrist. As you open the curtain, breathe out. Your head follows the general direction of the movement just enough to enable you to gaze beyond your hand (do not focus on it or you may become dizzy).

3 Turn your left palm downward and then bring your hand in a curve down to waist level. Continue the movement and bring your hand up to the point where it started, up beside your head. As your hand travels through this arc, breathe in. Follow the movement with your head, keeping your gaze just beyond your hand. Make between 10 and 30 circles with your left hand and then the same with your right hand.

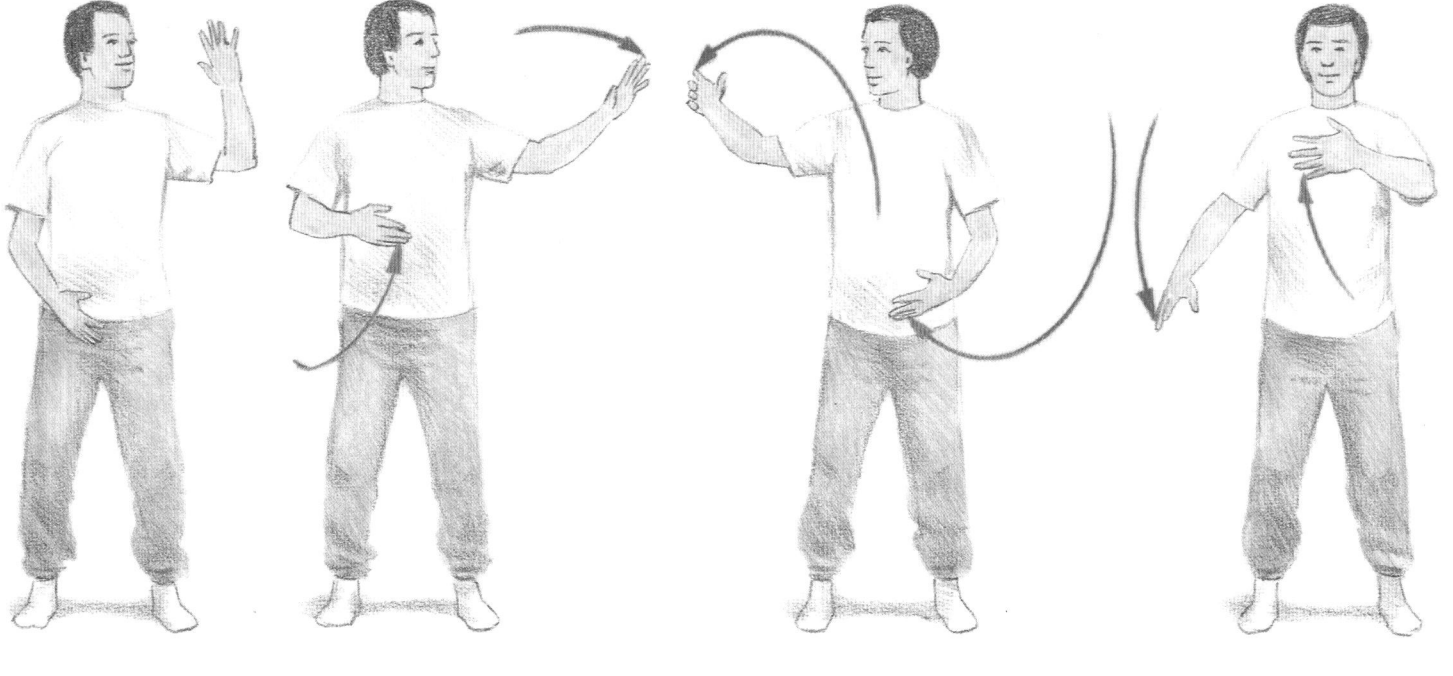

EXERCISE 24   WAVING HANDS LIKE CLOUDS

1   The aim of this exercise is to make the movement of the previous exercise, Opening the Curtain, simultaneously with both hands. To start, stand in the Wu Chi position with your knees slightly bent. Hold your left hand up beside your head, the palm facing outward, with the fingers gently spread. Hold your right hand near waist level, the palm facing the body.

2   Move your left hand over to the left as if you were opening a curtain. Your head follows the general direction of your hand. Continue the movement of your left hand downward in a curve to waist level. At the same time, scoop your right hand up to beside your head and turn the palm outward.

3   Now turn your head to let your gaze loosely follow the movement of your right hand as it circles outward and down toward the right. At the same time, your left hand comes in toward your body and then scoops up to beside your head and turns outward.

4   When you are comfortable with these movements, make the circles continuous. Imagine the palms of your hands are clouds drifting by you in the distant sky. Breathe naturally and keep the movement slow. Make a minimum of 10 circles and then build up to 30.

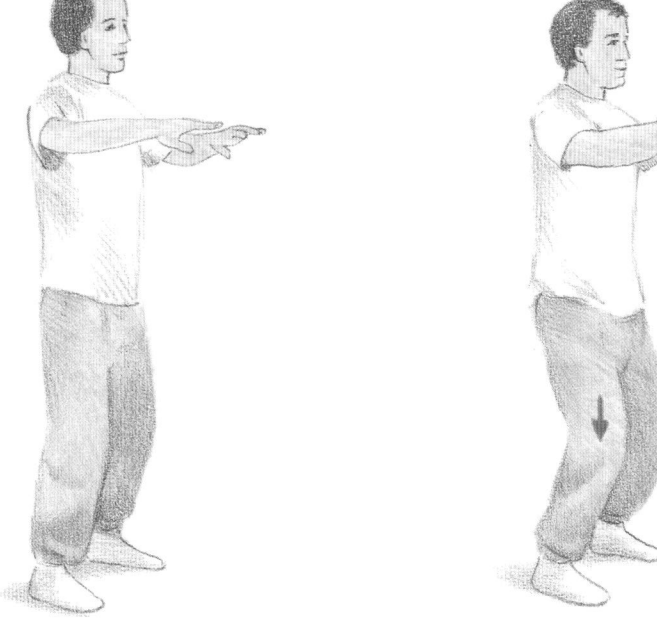

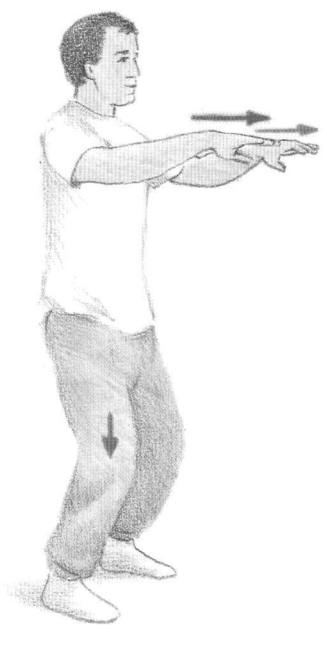

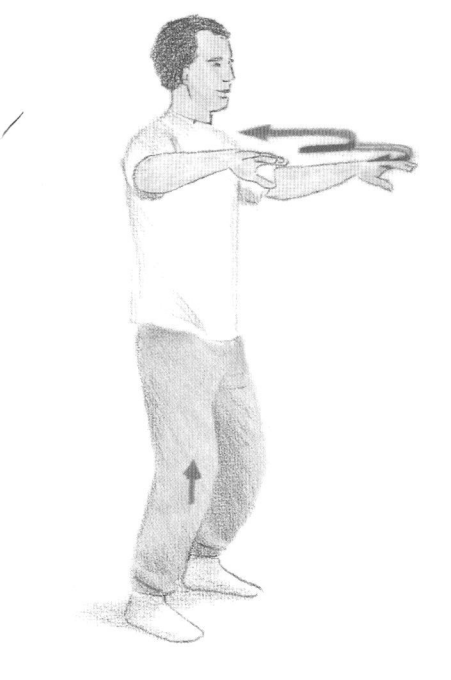

EXERCISE 25   SWIMMING IN DEEP WATER

1 This exercise is similar to Swimming on Land (*see p.27*), but with an important difference. To start, stand in the Wu Chi position with your knees slightly bent. Raise your hands gently up to chest height as if you were about to begin to swim using the breast-stroke. Breathe in.

2 Extend your arms forward as if you were moving ahead in the water and bend your knees to sink down. Keep the movement very smooth and calm. As your arms move forward and you sink down, breathe out. Keep your gaze directed forward with your head up.

3 Complete the breast-stroke movement by bringing both hands back toward your chest in gentle circles. At the same time, straighten your knees enough to rise up to the starting position where they were only slightly bent. Breathe in as your hands come back to your chest and you rise upward. Try to keep your body upright at all times and do not lean forward too much. Make a minimum of 10 complete strokes and try to work up to 30.

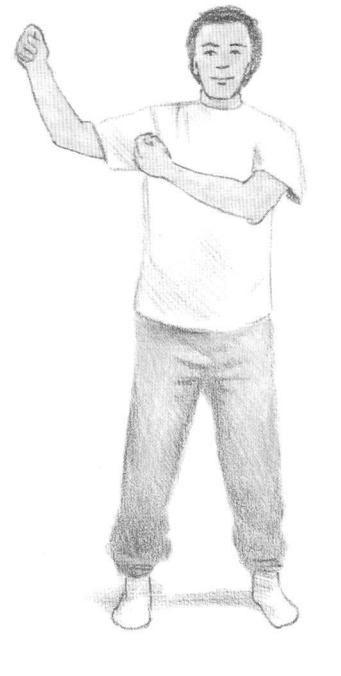
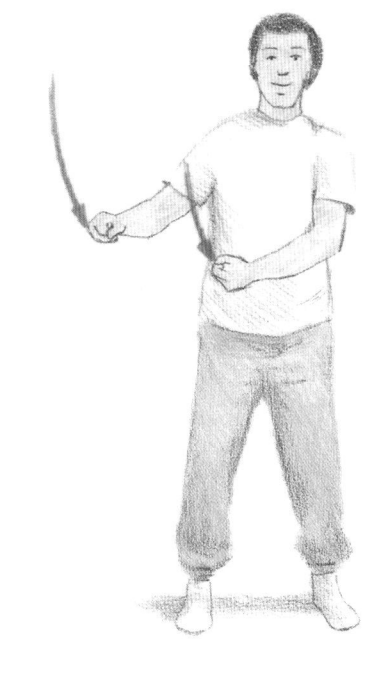
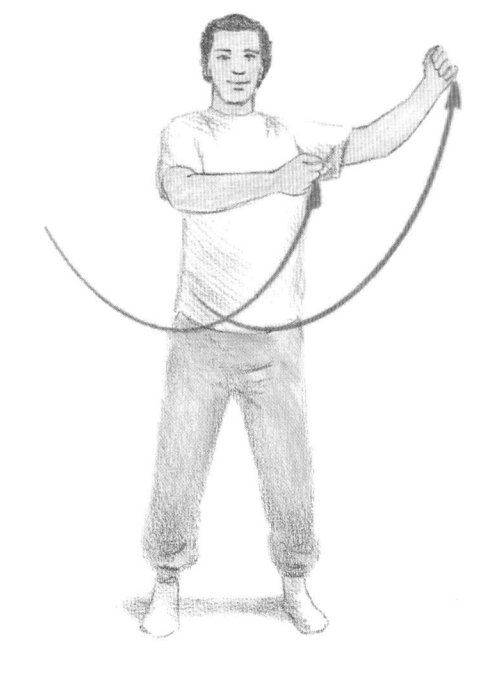

EXERCISE 26   SWEEPING FROM SIDE TO SIDE

1 Stand in the Wu Chi position with your knees slightly bent. Raise your right hand out to the side until it is level with your shoulder. Lift your left hand across your body so that it is opposite your right shoulder. Form very loose fists with your hands. Relax your shoulders. Breathe in.

1◆ *Fold your hand into a loose fist, as if holding an egg.*

2 Swing both arms down together and sweep them across in front of your body so that they swing up naturally to the other side, reaching shoulder or even head height. Breathe out strongly as the arms sweep down and across. This is a rapid, relaxed movement, as if your arms were suddenly released from a great height, swinging down and up with momentum.

3 Always breathe out as the arms sweep down and across. (You may not always feel the need to breathe in at the top of the sweep, but always breathe out on the downward motion.) When your arms reach the natural height of the upward movement, sweep them down and back across to the other side. Make a minimum of 10 sweeps, and up to 30 sweeps if you wish.

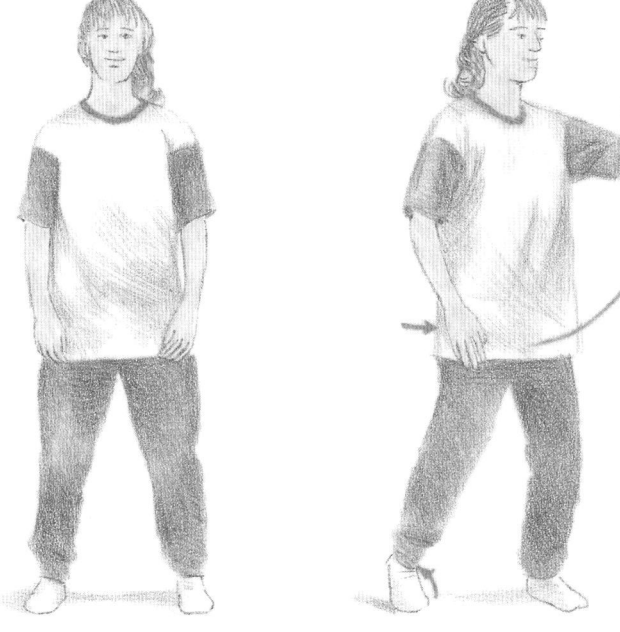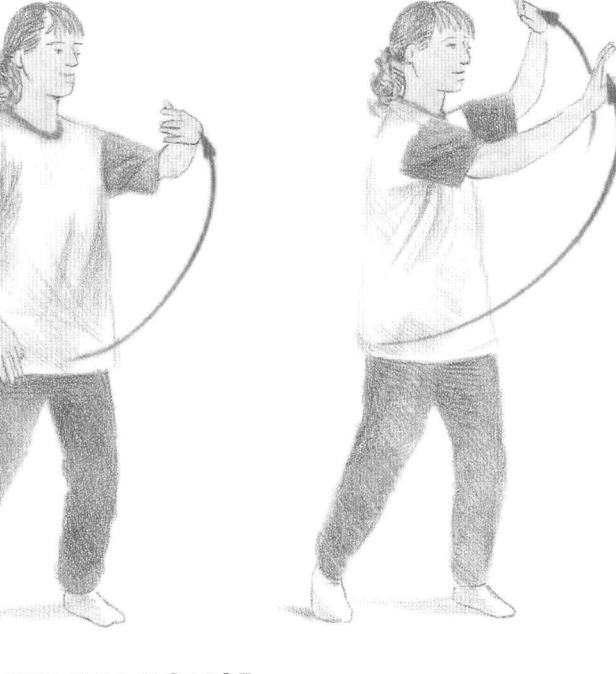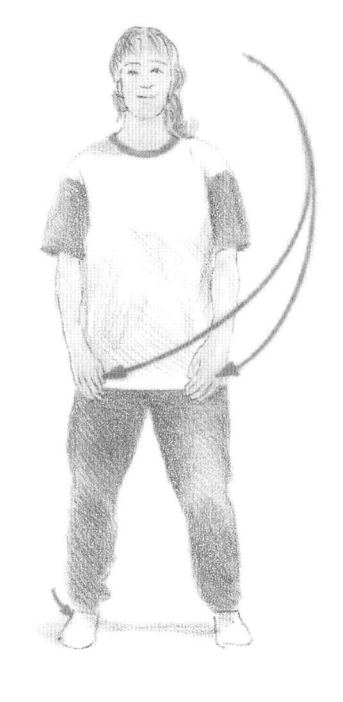

EXERCISE 27 BLOCKING TO THE DIAGONAL

1 Stand in the Wu Chi position, with your knees slightly bent and with your arms hanging loosely at your sides. Breathe in.

2 Raise your right heel off the ground and use the ball of your right foot to push your weight over to your left foot. As you do this, swivel a little to the left on the ball of your right foot, causing your body to turn in the same direction. At the same time, start to raise your left forearm up in an outward arc.

3 Continue the movement of your left forearm up to head height, and turn the palm outward. As you do this your right hand comes up and pushes slightly forward at chest height toward the left diagonal. Breathe out as your arm move.

4 Return to the starting position with your weight centered over both feet. Your knees are still slightly bent. Rest the palms of your hands lightly on your thighs. As you return to this position, breathe in. Repeat the full movement to the other side, so that your hands and face point to the right diagonal. Make between 10 and 30 of these complete movements to either side.

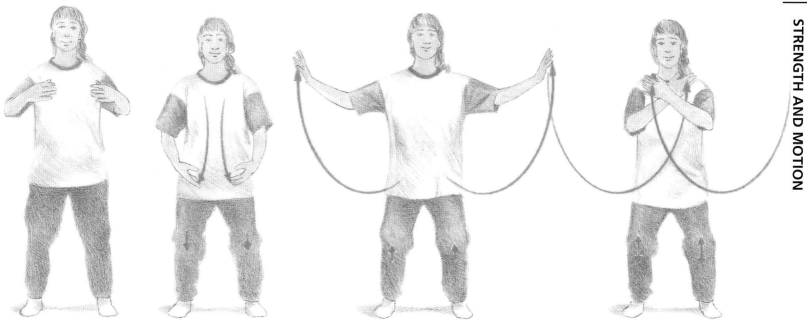

EXERCISE 28   EAGLE SPREADS ITS WINGS

1 Stand in the Wu Chi position and raise both of your arms up in front of you to chest height, as if you were holding a balloon between your arms and your chest. Breathe in.

2 Sweep both your arms down to hip level and, at the same time, bend your knees so that you sink slightly down. Start breathing out.

3 Continue the sweep of your arms rapidly out to the sides as if they were the spreading wings of an eagle. At the end of the movement, let your fingers open outward. As your arms are outward, your knees straighten up again, giving the effect of a gentle bounce as your arms make the full motion. Exhale completely.

4 Once your arms have fully extended there will be a natural recoil. Let both arms sweep rapidly back down and come up in front of your chest. It does not matter which hand is outermost. At the same time, breathe in. Your knees bend as your arms come down, and straighten up again as your arms cross in front of your chest, giving the effect of another bounce. Make 10 of these movements initially, increasing up to 30 as you improve.

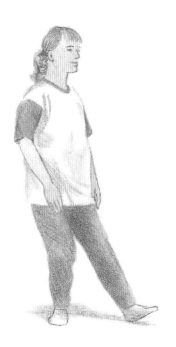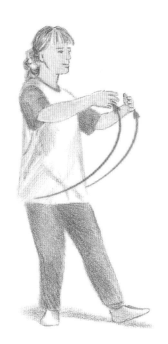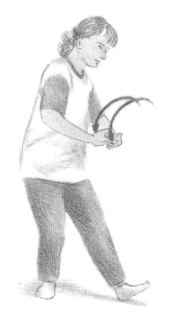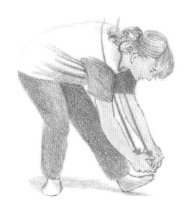

EXERCISE 29   BENDING FORWARD AND STRETCHING BACK

1 Start in the Wu Chi position, with your knees slightly bent, and shift your weight over to your right foot. Turn your body to the left diagonal and extend your left foot forward so that only the heel is resting lightly on the ground.

2 Raise both your arms up in front of you to chest height, as if you were holding a balloon between your arms and your chest. Breathe in. Hold that position for one second.

3 Breathe out as you bring your hands gently in toward your chest. Bend at the waist.

4 Extend your hands down toward the toes of your left foot. Go down only as far as you can without straining. Hold that position for one second.

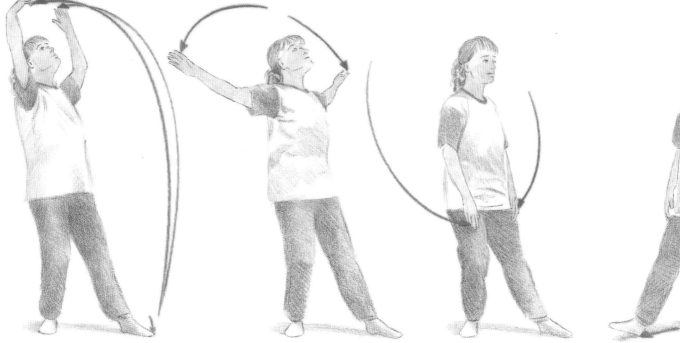

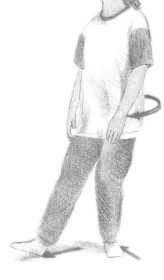

5 Breathe in as you come completely up, with your hands extended in front of you until they are above your head. Continue the movement as you carefully arch backward. Lower the toes of your left foot back down to the ground. Keep your weight on your right foot.

6 When you have arched back as far as you can without straining, gently turn your palms outward. Hold that position for one second.

7 Breathe out as you lower your arms to your sides and straighten your back. Hold that position for one second.

8 Move your left foot back to its start position and shift your weight on to it. Turn to the right diagonal and extend your right foot so that the heel rests on the floor. Raise both arms up in front of your chest as if you were holding a balloon between your arms and chest. Breathe in. Hold that position for one second. Then make the bending and stretching movement to that side. Make between 10 and 30 complete bends and stretches.

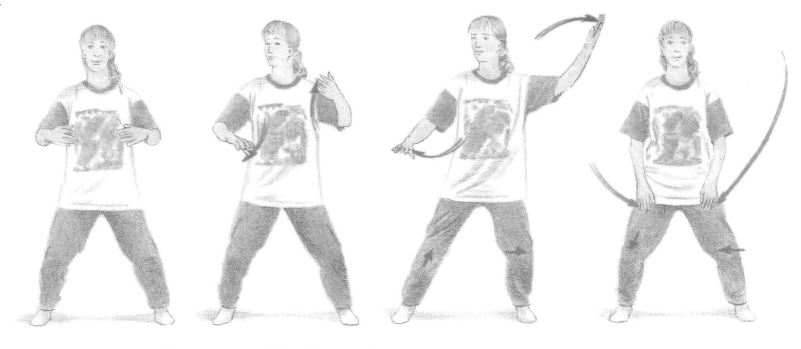

EXERCISE 30 THE MARE PARTS ITS MANE

1 Starting in the Wu Chi position, change the distance between your feet so that it is double the width of your shoulders. Your knees are bent and you are, accordingly, sitting down lower. Raise both hands in front of your belly as if you are holding a balloon.

2 Begin to move your hands apart. Your left hand sweeps out and up to the upper left diagonal with your palm facing upward. Your right hand slices down to the lower right diagonal with your palm facing downward.

3 As your hands separate, look to the right side. At the same time, transfer your weight over to your left foot and let your body lean a little in that direction. As you make the movement, breathe out.

4 Bring both hands in to rest on your thighs. Transfer your weight so that it is centered over both of your feet. Turn your head to face forward. Breathe in. Then repeat the sweeping movement to the other side, right hand up, left hand down, breathing out. Make a minimum of 10 sweeps, increasing to 30 as you improve.

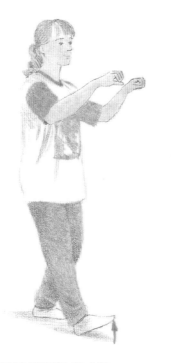
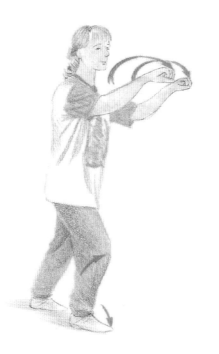
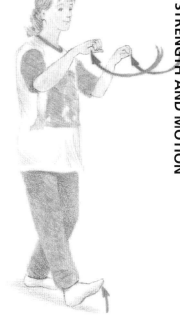

EXERCISE 31 **WORKING THE OAR**

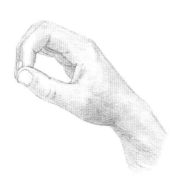

1 Stand with your feet shoulder-width apart. Move your right foot forward so that the space between your right heel and left toes is equal to the length of one of your feet. Raise both hands to chest height as if you were about to work an oar.

1♦ *Make loose fists as if you were holding an egg in each hand. Your thumbs rest lightly against your index fingers. Your elbows are slightly bent.*

2 Transfer your weight forward on to your right foot, until you feel that about three-quarters of your weight is on that foot. Be careful not to move your front knee beyond your toes. Your hands extend forward as you work the oar. As you make this movement, breathe out.

3 Then transfer your weight backward on to your left foot, until you feel that about three-quarters of your weight is on that foot. As you come back, slightly lift the ball of your right foot off the floor. Your arms come back as the weight shifts. As you make this movement, breathe in. Practice this movement at least 30 times with the right foot forward, then with the left one forward. Do more if you wish.

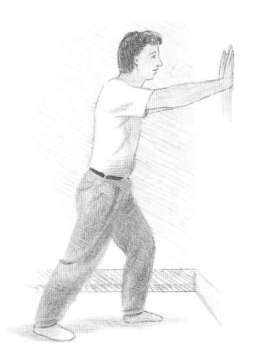 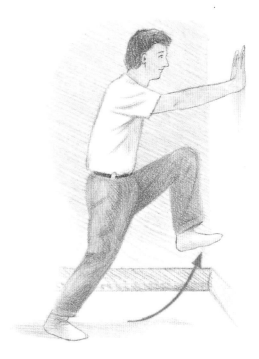

EXERCISE 32   PUSHING THE WALL

1 Stand facing a wall. Rest both of your hands against the wall at chest height. Your elbows should be bent a little. Step back with your right foot as far as you can, but keep your heel on the ground.

2 Keeping your palms securely pressed against the wall and your weight on your rear foot, lift your left knee up as high as you can. Feel as if you are pushing against the wall as hard as you can in a straight line running from the sole of your right foot up through to both your palms. Look straight ahead at the wall. Breathe out as you push. When you need to breathe in, relax slightly, but keep your left knee up. Then, press against the wall again as you breathe out. Complete between 10 and 30 presses on each leg.

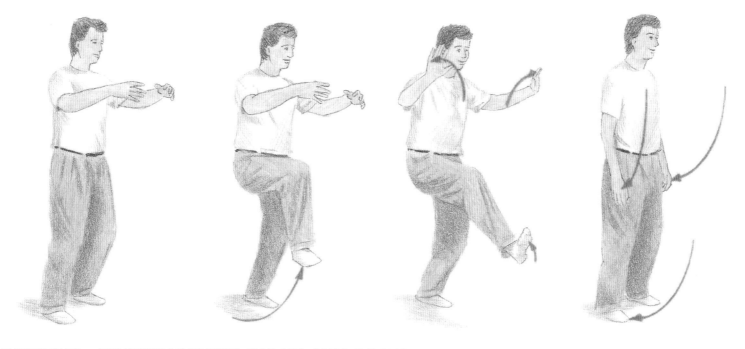

EXERCISE 33 SHOWING YOUR PALMS AND SOLES

1 Start in the Wu Chi position, with your knees slightly bent, and shift your weight over to your left foot. Raise your hands to chest height as if you were holding a large balloon between your hands. Start to breathe in.

2 Gently raise your right knee to the level of your waist. Finish breathing in.

3 Turn both of your palms outward and slightly extend your foot forward, as if you were pressing outward with your heel. As you do this, angle your foot slightly outward. Breathe out. Hold this position for one second.

4 Lower your right foot back down to the floor and bring your hands down to your sides. Center your weight equally over both of your feet. Breathe in and then out. Shift your weight to the right side, start to breathe in, and repeat the movement raising your left foot. Complete between 10 and 30 of these movements.

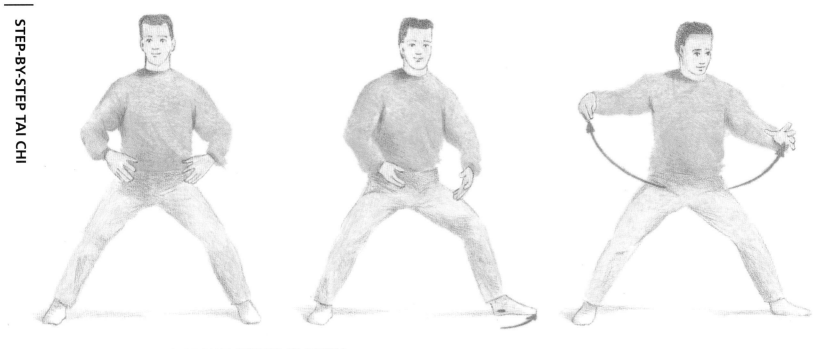

EXERCISE 34   SINGLE WHIP DOWN

1 Starting in the Wu Chi position, change the distance between your feet so that it is double the width of your shoulders. Raise your hands in front of you as if you were holding a balloon in front of your abdomen.

2 Swivel your left foot on its heel so that it points toward the left diagonal.

3 Make a "hook" with your right hand. (Do this by gently squeezing the pads of your fingertips against the pad of the tip of your thumb. Turn your wrist so that your fingertips and thumb point downward.) Extend it out a little to the right side. Extend your left arm out to the side also, with your left hand angled outward at about 45 degrees.

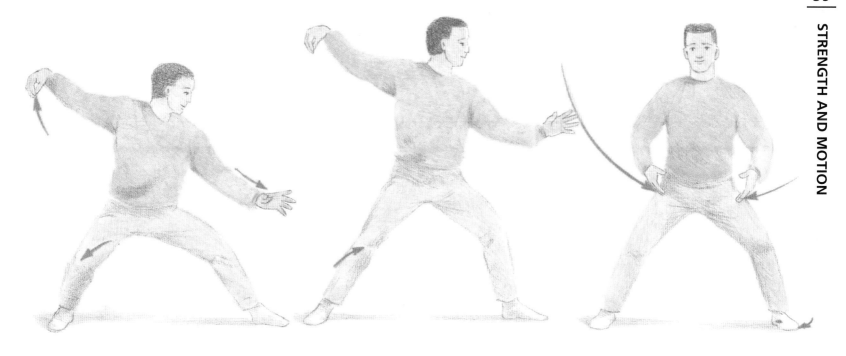

4 Transfer your weight over to your right foot and lower yourself as far as you can on that side, taking more of your weight on to your right leg. Breathe out as you sink down. Try to keep your torso upright. As you sink down, your right hand rises up level with your ear, and your left hand extends out to the side.

5 Straighten your right leg a little so that you rise up – but do not fully straighten it. Breathe in as you do this.

6 Bring both of your hands back in front of your abdomen to the starting position. Swivel on your left heel so that your foot faces forward again. Breathe out as you do this. Then, to do the exercise to the other side, swivel your right foot on its heel so it points to the right diagonal. Make a "hook" with your left hand, extend your right hand to the side, and repeat the movement with the weight shifting to the left. Make up to 10 of these movements to begin with and gradually increase to 30.

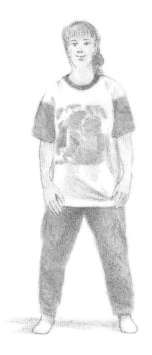 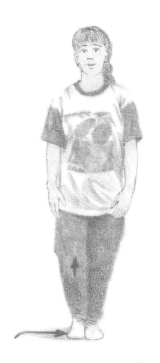 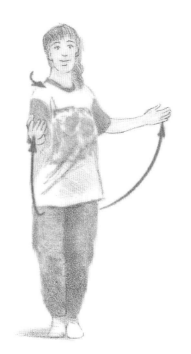 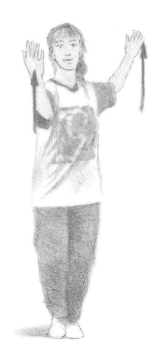

EXERCISE 35   MONKEY HOLDS THE WORLD

1 Start in the Wu Chi position with your knees bent and with your hands hanging loosely at your sides.

2 Shift your weight over to your left foot. Lift your right foot slightly off the ground and place the ball of your right foot lightly down beside the instep of your left foot.

3 Raise your arms up as if you were holding a huge globe.

3a Keep your head facing forward, but turn your shoulders so that your right arm comes up in front of your face and your left arm rises up to the back. The fingers of both hands are directed naturally upward. Breathe in as you raise your arms.

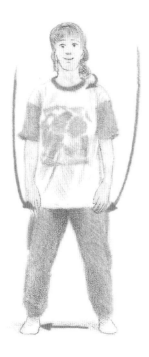

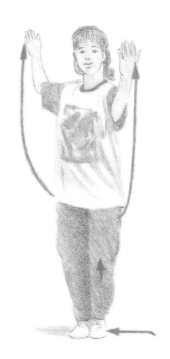

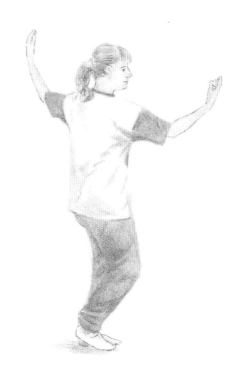

4 Lower your arms down to your sides and move your right foot back to the starting position, keeping your knees bent all the time. Center your weight over both of your feet. Breathe out as you make this return movement.

5 Now shift your weight to your right foot. Lift your left foot slightly off the ground and place the ball of your left foot lightly down beside the instep of your right foot.

6 Repeat the full sequence to this side. Make a minimum of 10 of these movements and progress up to 30 if you wish.

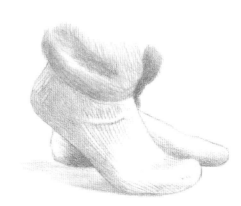

5◆ *The ball of your foot rests lightly on the ground beside the instep of the foot that bears your full weight.*

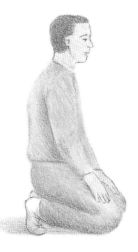

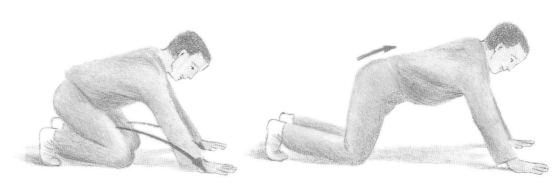

EXERCISE 36   STRETCHING LIKE A CAT

1 Kneel on the floor, resting your buttocks on your heels. Your feet are together and your toes are curled under. Relax your hands on your thighs.

2 Slowly rock forward so that you can place both your palms fully on the floor, as far forward as possible. Start to breathe out as you do this.

3 Continue to breathe out as you rock forward, raising your buttocks and shifting more of your weight forward.

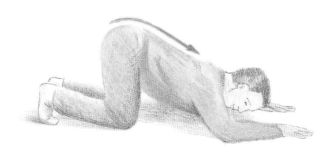

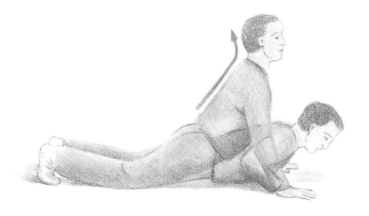

4 Keeping your hands and buttocks still, dip downward like a cat so that your chest nearly touches the floor. Look downward as you do this. Finish breathing out.

5 As you start to breathe in, gently arch your back and lift your head up.

6 Follow through so that your arms can straighten and your whole back is arched. Then come back to the original kneeling position and repeat this complete movement up to 10 times. Gradually increase to 30 times if you wish.

EXERCISE ROUTINES

There are three ways in which you can practice these advanced movements: you can treat all 18 of them as a sequence; you can practice them as individual exercises; or you can combine them according to your particular needs.

If you have just reached the point where you have become comfortable with Level 3 of the fundamental movements in Chapter One, you can now move on to doing these 18 instead. To begin with, perform each one three times and then pause – just as you did in the fundamental movements – before going on to the next new one. In total, these exercises should take you less than 10 minutes to complete.

If you are already familiar with Tai Chi movements, or have a sense of which movements would be of particular benefit to you, then simply select those ones from this chapter and perform them as often as you wish. If you would rather have a regular exercise routine, however, you can choose a small selection of the movements, changing the selection every month if you wish, to create your own programme of exercise. Two sample routines are given on the chart opposite as guidance.

There is one position you should always include in your routine, however: standing in the Wu Chi position. Even when you go on to learn the Small Circle Form, you should begin your work on the Form by standing in this position for two to three minutes.

EXERCISE ROUTINE 1	Level 1	Level 2	Level 3
	Length of time		
Exercise 19 Standing in Wu Chi	2 min	3 min	3 min
	Number of repetitions		
Exercise 20 Polishing the desk	10 each way	20 each way	30 each way
Exercise 22 Turning the balloon	10	20	30
Exercise 25 Swimming in deep water	10	20	30
Exercise 29 Bending forward and stretching back	10	20	30
Exercise 31 Working the oar	30	30	30
Exercise 33 Showing your palms and soles	10	20	30

EXERCISE ROUTINE 2	Level 1	Level 2	Level 3
	Length of time		
Exercise 19 Standing in Wu Chi	2 min	3 min	3 min
	Number of repetitions		
Exercise 21 Rolling the balloon	10 each way	20 each way	30 each way
Exercise 24 Waving hands like clouds	10	20	30
Exercise 30 The mare parts its mane	10	20	30
Exercise 31 Working the oar	30	30	30
Exercise 32 Pushing the wall	10 each side	20 each side	30 each side
Exercise 35 Monkey holds the world	10	20	30

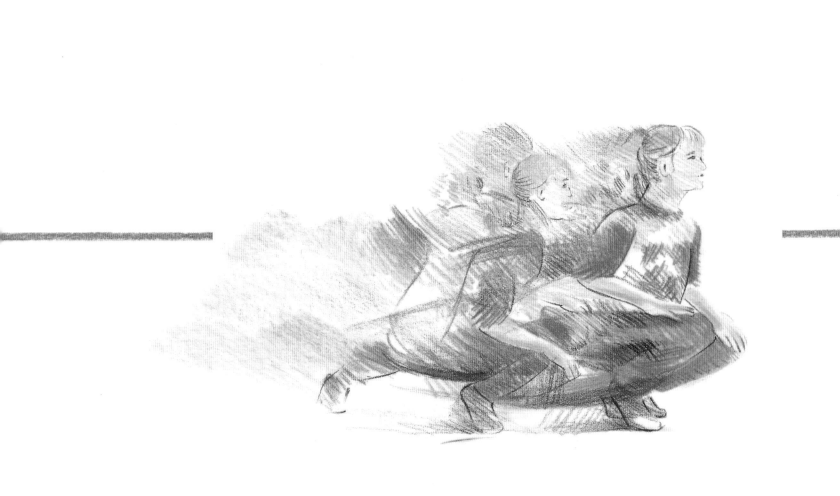

CHAPTER THREE

BALANCE AND MOVEMENT

The eight exercises in this chapter concentrate on stillness and movement. The first six develop your balance and ability to be still. The final two exercises – Tai Chi Walk and Duck Walk – are vital in teaching you to cultivate and control your balance while moving.

Balance is essential to Tai Chi. To begin with, simply being able to keep your balance is important to prevent falls and perhaps injuries. But having a good kinetic sense of balance means more than that: it is a manifestation of your inner balance – the health of your internal organs and the state of your nervous system. Not surprisingly, the idea of balance lies at the heart of Chinese medicine and philosophy. Because the outer and the inner are two aspects of the same quality of being, exercises that work at developing your physical balance can have a subtle healing effect on the balance of your internal chemistry as well.

At the same time, the patient work you put into these exercises strengthens the muscles in the lower part of your body. The exercises do this in a way very different to body building, however. You won't, for example, end up with bulging thigh or calf muscles, but their concealed strength will make them as powerful as steel springs.

As you practice you will develop many of the qualities needed for Tai Chi: balance, muscle control, concentration, and deep strength. Always keep your upper body relaxed. Move like a swan: effortless above the water, moving with strength below. Eventually you will see that these exercises have a profound quality. On the outside you are moving; on the inside you are still.

This inner stillness develops what we call "rooting" – a quality of being deeply connected to the earth, unshakeable and calm. Your whole body will become less tense in daily life, you will be more confident in yourself, and your spirit will move like a broad river.

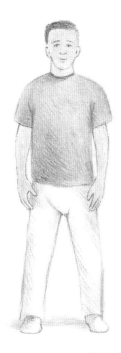
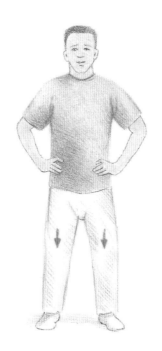
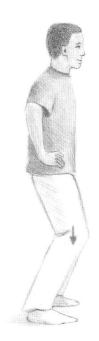

EXERCISE 37   HORSE RIDING STANCE

1 Begin in the Wu Chi position, with your feet facing forward, shoulder-width apart. Your hands hang loosely by your sides, and your shoulders are relaxed. Breathe naturally.

2 Rest your hands on your hips. Gradually bend your knees, lowering your backside as if you were starting to sit down on a chair. Lower yourself about 4 inches (10cm). If you cannot go that low to begin with, then gradually work toward that goal.

3 Your head remains upright. Make sure that your shoulders are relaxed and that you breathe naturally. Hold this position for three minutes. Once you are able to do that, you can extend the time period.

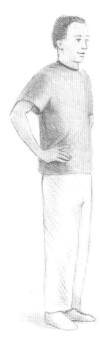
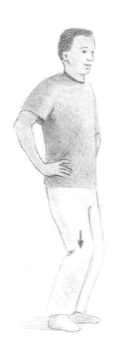
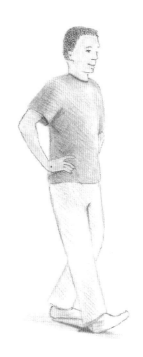

EXERCISE 38   SOFT STEP

1 Begin by standing upright with your heels together and your toes pointing slightly outward, forming a 45-degree angle. Rest your hands comfortably on your hips.

2 Gradually bend your knees, lowering your backside as if you were starting to sit down, keeping your heels together. Lower yourself about 4 inches (10cm). If you cannot go that low to begin with, then gradually work toward that goal.

3 Transfer your weight over to your left foot. Extend your right foot forward as if you were starting to step straight out, and lightly rest your right heel on the ground. Your head remains upright. Make sure that your shoulders are relaxed and that you breathe naturally. Work up to holding this position on each leg for three minutes – longer than this for intense training.

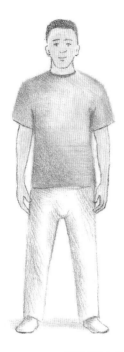

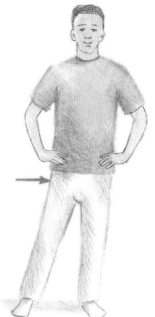

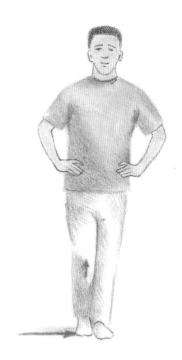

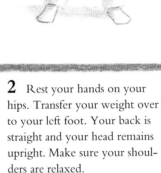

EXERCISE 39 STORK STEP

1 Begin in the Wu Chi position, with your feet facing forward, shoulder-width apart. Your hands hang loosely by your sides, and your shoulders are relaxed. Breathe naturally.

2 Rest your hands on your hips. Transfer your weight over to your left foot. Your back is straight and your head remains upright. Make sure your shoulders are relaxed.

3 Lift your right foot slightly off the ground and bring it over to your left foot, so that the ball of your right foot rests lightly on the ground beside the instep of your left foot. Your knees are nearly touching each other. Breathe naturally. Work up to holding this position on each leg for three minutes – longer for more intense training.

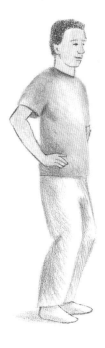
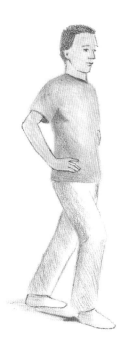
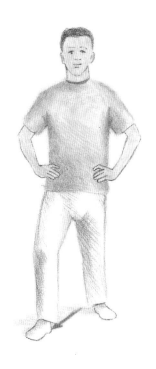

EXERCISE 40 BOW STEP

1 Begin by standing upright with your heels together and your toes pointing slightly outward, forming a 45-degree angle. Rest your hands on your hips. Gradually bend your knees, lowering your backside as if you were starting to sit down, keeping your heels together. Lower yourself about 4 inches (10cm). If you cannot go that low to begin with, then gradually work toward that goal.

2 Keep your left foot flat on the floor as you take a full step forward with your right foot, placing it flat on the floor in front of you. Transfer about three-quarters of your weight forward, careful not to extend your knee over your toes. Your bent front leg is the archer's bow. Your rear leg is the string for the arrow. Keep it reasonably straight but do not lock your knee.

3 Your back remains straight and your head is upright. Look straight ahead. Make sure that your shoulders are relaxed. Breathe naturally. Work up to holding this position with each leg forward for three minutes – longer for more intense training.

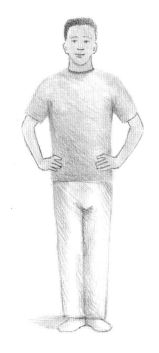

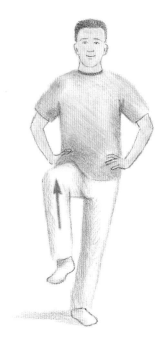

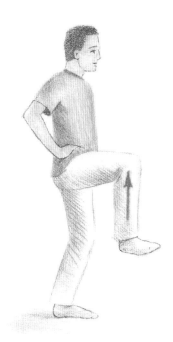

EXERCISE 41   COCKEREL STEP

1 Begin by standing upright with your heels together and your toes pointing slightly outward, forming a 45-degree angle. Rest your hands comfortably on your hips.

2 Transfer your weight over to your left foot. Raise your right knee so that it is level with your waist.

3 Your back is straight. Your head remains upright. Look straight ahead and make sure that your shoulders are relaxed. Breathe naturally. Work up to holding this position for three minutes on each leg – longer for more intense training.

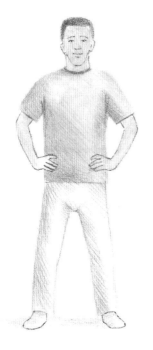
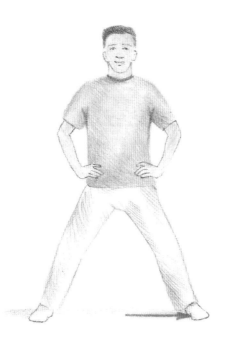
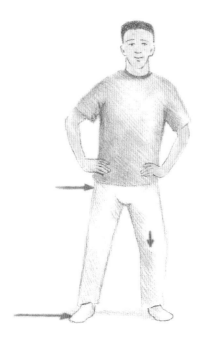

EXERCISE 42   SIDE STEP

1 Begin in the Wu Chi position, knees bent, with your feet facing forward, shoulder-width apart. Rest your hands on your hips. Your shoulders are relaxed. Breathe naturally.

2 Transfer your weight over to your right foot. Lift your left foot slightly and move it sideways so that the distance between your feet becomes twice the width of your shoulders.

3 Transfer your weight on to your left foot. Lift your right foot and move it toward your left foot so that the distance between your feet becomes the width of your shoulders. Your back is straight and your head upright. Look straight ahead. Your shoulders are relaxed. As you place each foot down, try to place all of the sole on the floor at the same time. Continue making these side steps in the space available. Reverse, moving to the right.

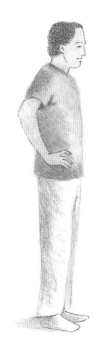
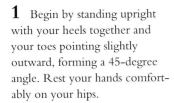
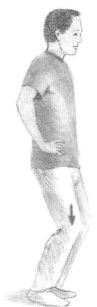
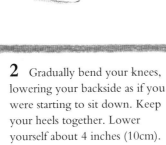
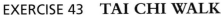
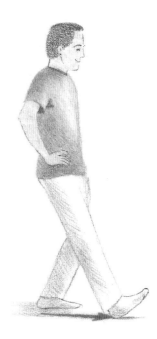

EXERCISE 43 TAI CHI WALK

1 Begin by standing upright with your heels together and your toes pointing slightly outward, forming a 45-degree angle. Rest your hands comfortably on your hips.

2 Gradually bend your knees, lowering your backside as if you were starting to sit down. Keep your heels together. Lower yourself about 4 inches (10cm).

3 Transfer your weight over to your left foot. Extend your right foot forward as if you were starting to step straight out, and lightly rest your right heel on the ground (*see the Soft Step, p.69*). As you make the step, breathe in.

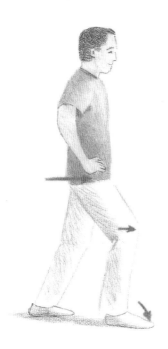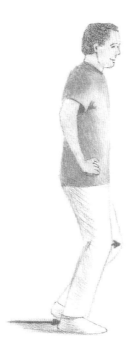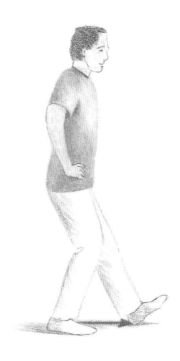

4 Place your right foot flat on the floor in front of you. Transfer about three-quarters of your weight forward, careful not to extend your knee past your toes (*see the Bow Step, p.71*). As your weight shifts forward, breathe out.

5 Transfer the rest of your weight forward to your right foot. Lift your left foot slightly off the ground and bring it up to your right foot, so that the ball of your left foot rests lightly on the ground beside the instep of your right foot. Your knees are nearly touching each other (*see the Stork Step, p.70*). As your rear foot comes forward, start to breathe in.

6 Extend your left heel forward and finish breathing in. Now continue the sequence of steps and matching breaths. Make all the movements as smoothly as possible. Make sure that your shoulders are relaxed and that your head remains upright. Keep your head level, as if you were carrying a saucer of water on it. Look straight ahead.

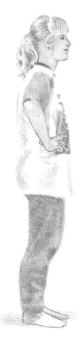
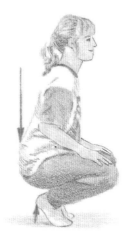
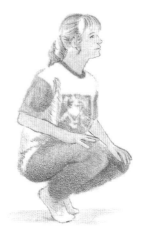
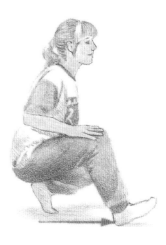

EXERCISE 44　DUCK WALK

1　Begin by standing upright, with your heels together and your toes pointing slightly outward, forming a 45-degree angle. Rest your hands comfortably on your hips.

2　Squat down so that your heels come off the ground and all your weight is on the balls of your feet. Rest your hands on your thighs.

3　Shift your weight over to the ball of your left foot and lower your left knee slightly.

4　Lift your right foot slightly off the ground and bring it forward so that you can place your right heel on the ground in front of you, in line with your left knee. (To do this, you must have all your weight firmly on the ball of your left foot.)

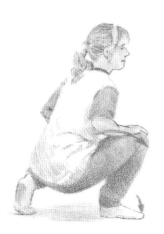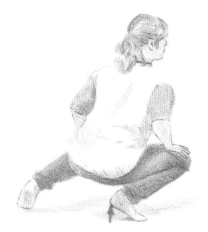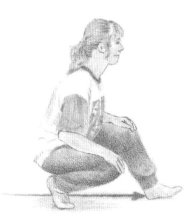

5 Lower the rest of your right foot on to the ground.

6 Transfer all of your weight forward from your left foot to your right foot. As you do this, roll forward so that your right heel comes up and all of your weight goes forward on to the ball of your right foot. Your hips will naturally swivel, turning your torso slightly to the left as you move.

7 Repeat the movement, starting by bringing your left foot forward so that you can place your left heel on the ground in front of you. Your hips turn naturally to the right with the movement. Keep practicing the walk in the space available.

Once you have mastered the movements, keep your back straight, your head upright, and look forward in order to maintain your balance.

EXERCISE ROUTINES

The key to performing these exercises correctly is perseverance in practice to develop endurance. In Tai Chi, this is achieved not by adopting a stiff body or an unyielding attitude, but rather through relaxation, acceptance and patience. Part of the art of Tai Chi is to learn how to develop these virtues under pressure. Some of the exercises in this chapter require you to hold a position without moving for several minutes. Those that involve no pain simply require patience. This is excellent training for your mind and your nerves – training that will be immensely helpful to you if you are suffering from stress.

Several of the stationary exercises do make strong demands on your muscles, however, and they can be painful to do. If the pain becomes unbearable and you are worried that you may injure yourself, then stop. (If you are recuperating from an illness or have a history of injury in that area, for example, you may wish to consult a doctor before trying these.) Otherwise, look on the pain as your teacher. Pay attention to it. Try to see which muscle group is affected. Then make a deliberate effort to tell those muscles to relax, without changing your position. This will call on and develop your inner qualities of acceptance, relaxation, and endurance.

The same advice applies to the two movement exercises, the Tai Chi Walk and the Duck Walk. Pay careful attention to each movement. Do not let your mind wander. Use the exercises to strengthen your sense of balance and do not be distracted from this essential work by any temporary sensations of pain.

Do the stationary exercises (37 – 41) separately from the rest of your Tai Chi practice. Choose one (each day or every week) and just practice standing still in that position at a convenient time in your day. (You can do exercises like this while waiting for a kettle to boil, or while reading a newspaper article, for example.)

You can add one of the moving exercises (42 – 44) at the end of your other Tai Chi exercise routines. If you do not have room to make all the steps in a straight line moving forward, you can go around in a gentle circle or square by rotating on the appropriate foot just enough to enable you to turn in whatever direction is necessary.

EXERCISE ROUTINE	Level 1	Level 2	Level 3
	Duration/number of repetitions		
Exercise 37 Horse riding stance	1.5 min	3 min	5 min
Exercise 38 Soft step	1 min each leg	2 min each leg	3 min each leg
Exercise 39 Stork step	1.5 min each leg	2 min each leg	5 min each leg
Exercise 40 Bow step	1.5 min each leg	3 min each leg	5 min each leg
Exercise 41 Cockerel step	1 min each leg	2 min each leg	3 min each leg
Exercise 42 Side step	10 steps	20 steps	30 steps
Exercise 43 Tai Chi walk	10 steps	20 steps	30 steps
Exercise 44 Duck walk	6 steps	12 steps	24 steps

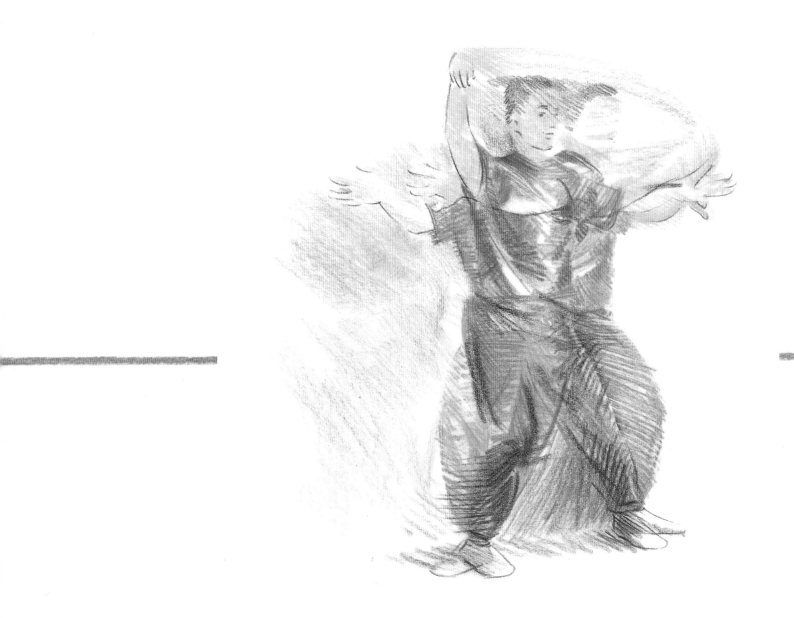

CHAPTER FOUR

WORKING WITH A PARTNER

This part of the book introduces you to a set of Tai Chi movements that you can practice with a partner. Ideally, both of you should have practiced the exercises in the first three chapters on your own before moving on to these movements. If you can only manage to do the movements in Chapter One, however, you can still experiment with two of the movements in this chapter – Sawing Wood and Polishing the Window.

Exercising with a partner has important advantages for both people concerned. First, it increases awareness and sensitivity, since both of you have to pay attention not only to ensuring that your own individual movements are smooth, but also to the subtle variations in the movements of the other person. And second, exercising with a partner makes your muscles and nerves more alert, and helps to develop a sense of harmony and timing.

Since these Tai Chi movements lead to a harmonious exchange of energy between two people, it is ideal to practice the exercises regularly with a friend or your partner. But if regular practice proves impossible, don't worry; even working together occasionally will help you to perform some of the most essential leg and hip movements needed in your Tai Chi form.

You will also discover that practicing these movements with a partner is a wonderful form of relaxation – even more so than doing the movements on your own. Of course, at first you may find that it requires more concentration to get the right balance of control, relaxation, and slow movement. After that, however, the results will be truly rewarding.

If both of you are learning Tai Chi, you can still practice these exercises together even if you are at different levels of study. Just practice individually in your own way and then come together at the end of the session to do some of these joint movements.

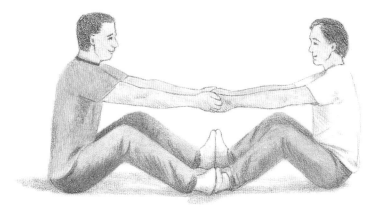

EXERCISE 45 ROWING THE BOAT

1 Sit facing each other with your legs spread apart, and with the soles of your feet touching. Reach toward each other and hook your fingers together.

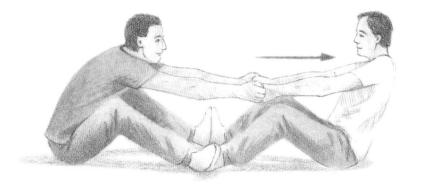

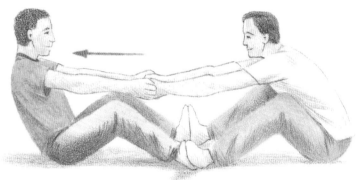

2 One of you leans back, breathing in. Both of you should keep your arms straight and move just your bodies. The backward lean naturally pulls the other person forward, and this person breathes out. Don't try to stretch your legs out straight or overdo the backward and forward movement. Just go as far as feels comfortable within the natural limits of your bodies.

3 When you have rowed in one direction, reverse direction. Complete six of these backward and forward movements. Then unhook your fingers and both slowly stand up.

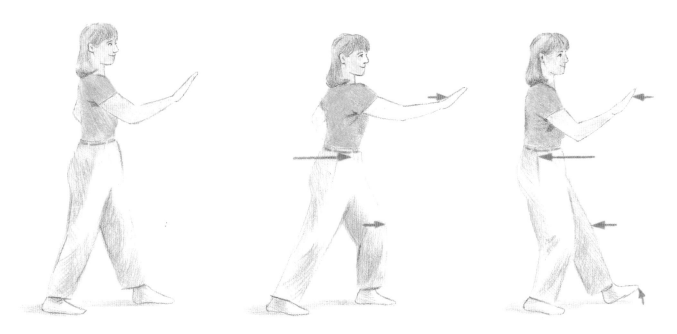

EXERCISE 46   SAWING WOOD

1 To begin with, each of you should practice the movement on your own. Stand with your feet shoulder-width apart. Move your left foot forward so that the space between your left heel and your right toes is equal to the length of one of your feet. Rest your left hand on your hip. Raise your right hand in front of you so that your outstretched palm is at chest level. Your wrist and elbow are slightly bent.

2 Transfer your weight forward on to your left foot, until you feel that about three-quarters of your weight is on that foot. Be careful not to move your front knee beyond your toes. Your right hand extends slightly forward as you shift your weight. Your elbow and wrist remain slightly bent. As you make this movement, breathe out.

3 Then transfer your weight backward on to your right foot, until you feel that about three-quarters of your weight is on that foot. As you come back, slightly lift the ball of your left foot off the floor. Your right arm comes slightly back as the weight shifts. As you make this movement, breathe in. Practice this movement until you feel comfortable with it. Try doing it at least 30 times. You can do more if you want. Now try it with your partner.

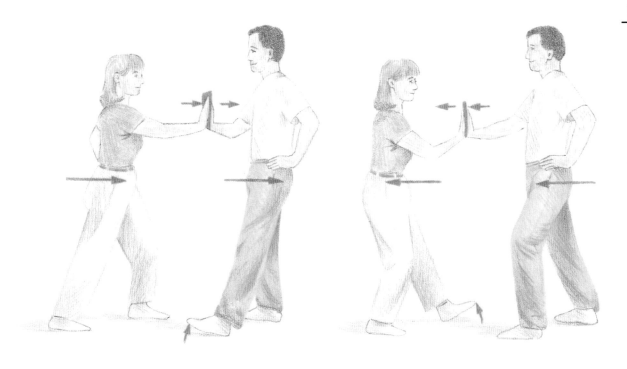

4 Face each other squarely in the starting position, so that the tips of the toes of your front feet are level with each other. Put your right palms together. Place a piece of paper or cardboard in between your hands and hold it lightly in position. Just as if you were using a two-handed saw, start to transfer your weight so that one person comes forward and the other person rocks backward. Be careful to keep your hands continually in contact so that the paper or cardboard does not fall.

5 When you have completed that motion, reverse the action. The person whose weight was forward now rocks backward, and the other person comes forward. As you make these movements, keep your bodies upright and avoid leaning forward or tilting backward. Synchronize your breathing with your movements. You can practice this exercise for as long as you like, but do a minimum of 30 backward and forward motions. You can also do this exercise with your right foot forward and your left hand up in front – both singly and as a couple.

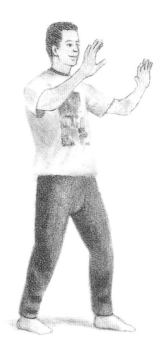 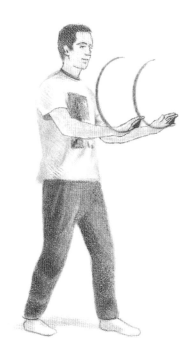 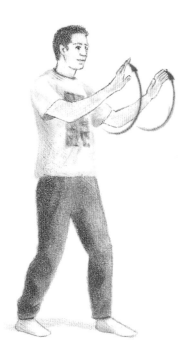

EXERCISE 47 POLISHING THE WINDOW

1 To begin with, each of you should practice these movements on your own. Stand with your feet shoulder-width apart. Move your left foot forward so that the space between your left heel and your right toes is equal to the length of one of your feet. Raise both of your hands in front of you so that your outstretched palms are level with your chest. Your wrists and elbows are slightly bent.

2 Move both of your hands in small clockwise circles (your hands circle first to the right). The movement should feel as if you are polishing a window with both of your hands. Breathe naturally.

3 Both your hands make large full circles on the flat "window" in front of you.

Then, when you have polished the window to the right, reverse the movement so that your hands circle to the left. Practice both these motions until you feel comfortable with them. Try doing each of them at least 30 times. You can do more if you want. Then go on to do this exercise with your partner.

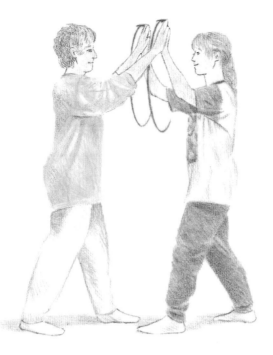 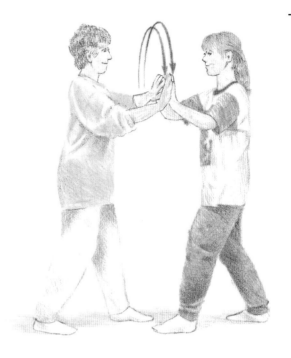

4 Stand facing each other squarely with your left feet in front, so that the tips of the toes of your front feet are level with each other. Put both of your palms together. Just as if you were polishing both sides of the window at the same time, make at least 30 clockwise circles. Be sure to keep your hands lightly pressed against each other. Keep your bodies still and upright.

5 When you have completed that movement, reverse direction. You can practice this exercise for as long as you like, but be sure to do a minimum of 30 movements with your hands moving in each direction.

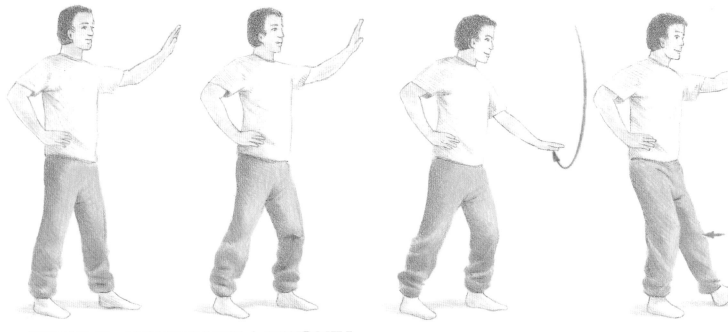

EXERCISE 48   MOVING LIKE A WINDMILL

1 To begin with, each of you should practice the movement on your own. Stand with your feet shoulder-width apart. Move your left foot forward so that the space between your left heel and your right toes is equal to the length of one of your feet. Rest your right hand on your hip. Raise your left arm so that it is fully outstretched at a 45-degree angle in front of your head.

2 Transfer your weight forward on to your left foot, until about three-quarters of your weight is on that foot. Be careful not to move your front knee beyond your toes.

3 Your left arm circles downward and to the left as you shift your weight forward. As you make this movement, breathe out.

4 Then transfer about three-quarters of your weight backward on to your right foot. Slightly lift the ball of your left foot. Your left arm continues the circle back up to head height. As you do so, breathe in. Practice the movement at least 30 times, both with your left foot and left arm forward, then with your right foot and right arm forward.

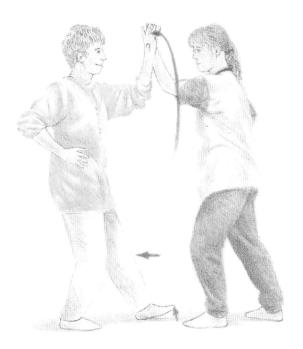

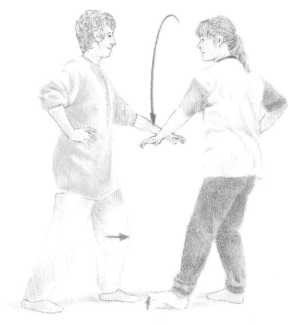

5 Face each other squarely so that the tips of the toes of your front feet are level with each other, and cross your left wrists.

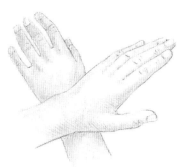

Transfer your weight so that as one person moves forward the other rocks backward. The one moving backward takes the other person's arm over to the left in a circle (*see opposite*), so that their wrist carries the other person's arm over to the left and down. The one moving backward should keep their wrist in constant contact with the other person's. This is known as "sticking".

5♦ *Cross your wrists so that they touch each other and remain lightly in contact as you both circle your arms.*

6 Both people's hands are now at the bottom of the circle. Then continue the circle upward. As you do this, the person whose weight was forward now rocks backward, and the other person comes forward. As you make these movements, keep your bodies upright and avoid leaning forward or tilting backward. Synchronize your breathing with your movements. You can practice this exercise as long as you like, but do a minimum of 30 circles leading both with the left hand and foot and then with the right hand and foot.

EXERCISE ROUTINES

The exercise routine below will help you work through the four movements to which you have been introduced in this chapter. Bear in mind that before attempting any of the last three exercises with a partner, you should first practice the basic movements on your own. This is important for developing the familiarity and balance with them that will allow you to relax as you work with your partner.

You can also add these exercises for two to the end of your individual exercise and Tai Chi practice sessions. Until you are comfortable with these movements, always start at Level 1 and work slowly and carefully. If you are only able to do the fundamental exercises in Chapter One, just try Sawing Wood and Polishing the Window.

WORKING WITH A PARTNER	Level 1	Level 2	Level 3
Movements			
	Duration or number of repetitions		
Exercise 45 Rowing the boat	6	9	12
Exercise 46 Sawing wood	30	45	60
Exercise 47 Polishing the window	30 each way	45 each way	60 each way
Exercise 48 Moving like a windmill	30 each way	45 each way	60 each way

TAI CHI FUNDAMENTALS: ROUTINE	Initial	Advanced
Movements	**Duration or number of repetitions**	
Exercise 19 Standing in Wu Chi	3 minutes	3 minutes
Exercise 1 Relaxing the neck	3 each way	6 each way
Exercise 5 Two full moons	6	12
Exercise 10 Bending forward	3	6
Exercise 14 Knee circles	15 each way	30 each way
Exercise 21 Rolling the balloon	15 each way	30 each way
Exercise 24 Waving hands like clouds	10	20
Exercise 25 Swimming in deep water	15	30
Exercise 28 Eagle spreads its wings	15	30
Exercise 29 Bending forward and stretching back	5 to each side	10 to each side
Exercise 41 Cockerel step	1.5 min each leg	3 min each
Exercise 43 Tai Chi walk	15 steps	30 steps
Exercise 44 Duck walk	12 steps	24 steps
Exercise 48 Moving like a windmill	15 each way	30 each way
Exercise 19 Standing in Wu Chi	1 minute	1 minute

This is a full routine based on the first part of the book. In the same way, you can create your own routine to meet your individual needs

PART 2

THE SMALL CIRCLE FORM

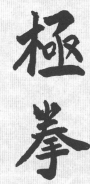

The slow and elegant exercise movements of Tai Chi are woven together into what we call a "form". Oddly enough, it is called a form because it is empty. It is you who fill the form.

What follows on these pages is a set of precise instructions that tell you, step-by-step, exactly how to make each of the movements in the Form. You will recognize many of them from the exercises in Part One. If you have been carefully practicing those exercises you will find that they have quietly laid a firm foundation for the balance and control needed to learn the Form.

This is the reason why it is so important to avoid the temptation to skip over the exercises and start directly on this part of the book. Tai Chi is a complete system. It must be learned in a careful and methodical fashion if you are to obtain the maximum possible benefit and avoid the possibility of injury.

The first stage is to learn each of the 15 movements in the Small Circle Form as meticulously as possible. You do this by breaking each one up into its smaller component parts. The result is that you begin by learning small, distinct motions, giving the impression that you are making slow mechanical actions rather like a robot. This is essential to ensure that you start off learning thoroughly the precise little elements of each main movement. In Chapter Six, you will learn how to connect up all the elements and produce beautiful flowing Tai Chi.

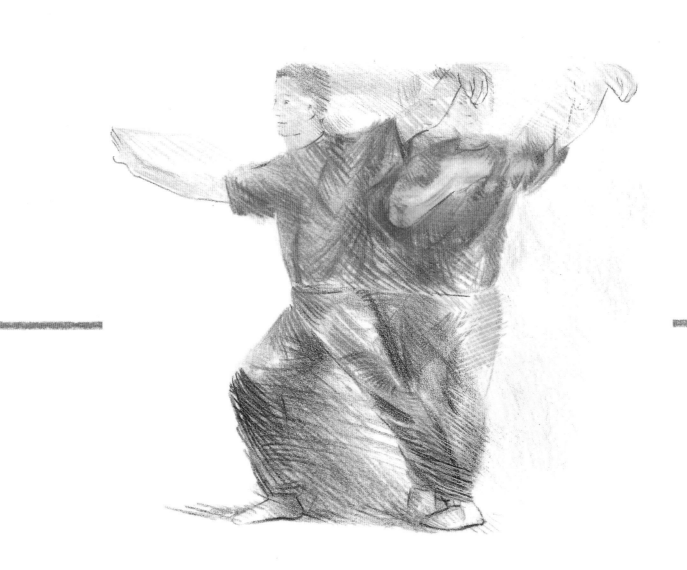

CHAPTER FIVE

The Form

The Small Circle Form is a smooth, flowing sequence of gentle movements. When you have learned it and practiced it for some time, it will take you about one and a half minutes to perform. But to be able to do it well, you will need to pay very careful attention to the precise instructions and illustrations that follow. Learn a little each week and concentrate on doing that well, rather than trying to speed ahead through the whole routine as quickly as possible.

Ideally, you should set aside about 20 to 30 minutes a day for your Tai Chi. You will need to keep up your Tai Chi exercise routine while you are learning the form, because the process of becoming supple and strong must continue. Then, after your exercises, work on learning the movements in the Form, reviewing and practicing what you have learned up to that point.

There are 15 main movements in the Small Circle Form. Each one has a name, such as Tai Chi Starting or Single Whip. You will find these names as bold headings throughout the following pages. To let you see the precise detail of each of these main movements, you are shown, step-by-step, the component parts. These are numbered consecutively from 1 to 75. So, for example, Tai Chi Starting comprises numbers 1 through 5. The next main movement begins at number 6 and so on.

One movement at a time

Usually, people are taught one main movement at a time. So, to begin, try to learn Tai Chi Starting. Start at number 1 and finish at number 5. Just try to learn that in your first week,

practicing with care every day. Then, when you have that firmly in mind, go on to the next main movement, Hold the Ball (numbers 6 to 11). Learn that over the course of the second week. Avoid rushing ahead. If you try to take in too much at a time, you won't learn the movements correctly, you won't remember them properly, and you may give up! Tai Chi is the one thing you must learn to take nice and easy. Just think that you are going to give yourself one Tai Chi class a week. Teach yourself one, and only one, main movement in that class, and then practice what you learned in that class throughout the week until the next class.

One important advantage of having this step-by-step book is that you can go back to check exact, detailed points at any time. A step-by-step learning routine for those with no previous Tai Chi experience is included on pages 124-5. This is followed by a summary of the main movements to help you remember the full sequence when you practice the complete Small Circle Form.

Working with this book

One problem you will come up against is the fact that you cannot learn and carry out the Tai Chi movements and hold a book at the same time! To overcome this, you could, for example, try propping the book up in front of you on something like a music stand or on a convenient shelf. Or you could ask a friend to hold the book and read it out aloud to you (you could try learning the form together, helping each other).

Try reading the instructions very, very slowly on to an audio tape and then play them back to yourself. You can also use a mirror to check that your positions correspond to the drawings

in the book. Don't assume that you will get everything right the first time. Just do your best to get the basic idea of the movements first and then go back to check and refine the details.

Repetition and learning

Repetition is part of Tai Chi. The movements must become automatic before you reach the relaxed, flowing stage. When you are teaching yourself, therefore, spend time first reading and experimenting with the movement that you are going to learn that week. Then repeat it at least nine times in silence, paying careful attention to what you are doing. Then read the instructions and look at the illustrations again. Next, correct yourself as you repeat the movement another nine times, and check once more and repeat. Don't give up if you find it difficult that day and don't stop early if it seems too easy for you. This is a subtle, refined system of personal development. Be patient and don't fall prey to messages of boredom, impatience, or frustration coming from your nervous system. They are the proof that you need the profound benefits of Tai Chi.

The learning is cumulative and each movement follows on from the previous one. Work at learning each new movement in your weekly "class", but when you are practicing over the rest of the week, review the whole of the form up to and including that movement as well. You may find that your legs tremble or that you are a little shaky. This is normal. The exercises in Chapter Three will help correct this, so be sure to include these in your exercise routine.

Some people ask "What should I think about when I am doing Tai Chi?" The answer for those who are learning the form at this stage is: "Think about what you are doing". It is so important to get the movements correct and this is what you should concentrate your whole

attention on. For example, make sure that you are moving your hands and feet into position exactly in the way described in the text and shown in the pictures. The discipline of learning Tai Chi correctly leads to great freedom. But the discipline of being correct comes first! When you complete your daily session, there is one thing that will contribute greatly to your whole development. Don't instantly rush off to get on with the next thing in your life. Instead, stand in the Wu Chi position for a minute. Just stand there, feet shoulder-width apart, hands loosely by the side. Nothing more. Then move forward into the rest of your day.

Understanding the instructions

Each component part of every main movement is shown by an illustration with its explanatory text. In the first half of the Small Circle Form, some of these components are further broken down into two stages, the second of which is marked with the letter "a". This is to help you see clearly a long motion such as the full sweep of an arm. Several small adjustments may be involved in each of these component parts and these are all described in the text. Each illustration shows the final position of your body after all the adjustments have been made.

To help you understand how your body moves into that position, arrows indicate the key movements. But they don't show all the resulting shifts in your position, only the actions on which you need to concentrate. For example, if you swivel on your foot, other parts of your body will move as well (your heel, calf, knee, hip, and so on). This occurs naturally. The text, illustration, and arrows tell you what basic movement to make, from which the rest will flow.

The directions

The instructions for the Form tell you which direction to face and where to turn or move your feet. These directions refer to an imaginary square (see below) in which you stand. The front of the square refers to the line of the square in front of you when you begin, facing forward. Other directions use the front as their reference point, regardless of which way your body has turned. For example, moving your hand to the "right diagonal" always refers to the right diagonal of the imaginary square. The path of a movement described in the text is shown on its accompanying illustration by an arrow. The figure itself shows the final position of the body, but the arrow's tail begins where each movement starts. In most cases, this corresponds precisely to the position of that part of the body in the previous picture.

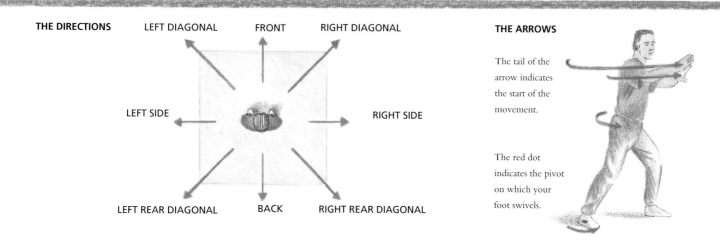

THE DIRECTIONS

LEFT DIAGONAL   FRONT   RIGHT DIAGONAL

LEFT SIDE   RIGHT SIDE

LEFT REAR DIAGONAL   BACK   RIGHT REAR DIAGONAL

THE ARROWS

The tail of the arrow indicates the start of the movement.

The red dot indicates the pivot on which your foot swivels.

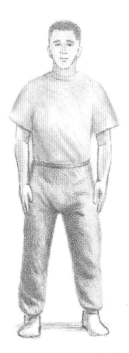

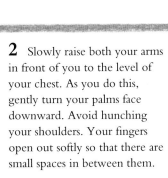

TAI CHI STARTING

All Tai Chi movement emerges out of stillness. Before you begin the Form, adopt the Wu Chi position (*see Exercise 19, p.42*). When you have completed this exercise, rise up until your knees are straight but not locked. Then begin the Tai Chi Form.

1 Stand straight with your feet shoulder-width apart. Check that your toes are pointing straight forward and that your knees are unlocked. Let your back hang straight down to the bottom of your spine. Relax your stomach muscles. Lower your shoulders and let your hands hang loosely by your sides. Face forward.

2 Slowly raise both your arms in front of you to the level of your chest. As you do this, gently turn your palms face downward. Avoid hunching your shoulders. Your fingers open out softly so that there are small spaces in between them.

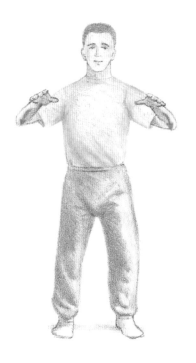

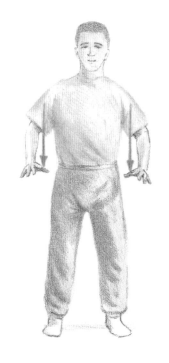

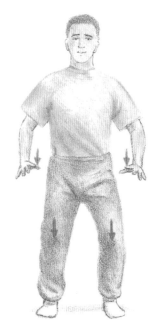

HOLD THE BALL (RIGHT)

3 Slowly lower your elbows so that both your hands are drawn half way back toward your chest. Your hands remain shoulder-width apart, level with your chest.

4 Lower both your hands in front of you to just below the level of your hip. Both palms are still facing downward.

4◆ *Your hands are close to your body in line with your hips. They are angled a little downward and turned slightly inward.*

5 Lower your backside as if you were slowly starting to sit straight down. Keep your lower back tucked in as you do this. Your knees bend slightly and your weight gradually shifts back a little.

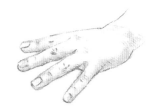

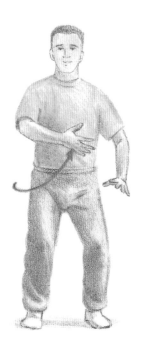
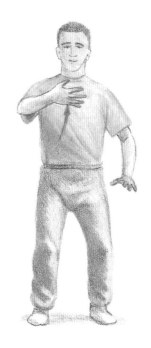
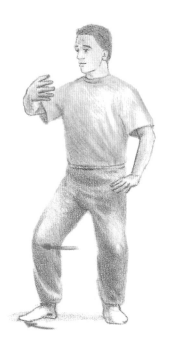
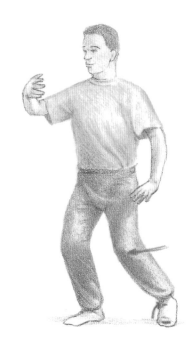

6 Slowly curve your right forearm up and out in front of your torso.

6a Continue until the center of your right palm reaches a point about a foot in front of the center of your chest. It is as if you were gently holding a large balloon between your forearm and your chest.

7 Keep your left foot in place. Carefully swivel on your right heel so that your right foot turns 45 degrees to the right. Your hips and upper body turn gently in the same direction.

8 Shift your weight forward on to the sole of your right foot while slightly raising your left heel. Swivel on the ball of that foot so that your left knee also turns a little to the right.

8◆ *Your right foot points to the right diagonal. Your left foot is turned in that direction also, but not fully. Although your upper body is now facing the right diagonal, this is due only to the slight change in your foot position. Your torso and right arm have not moved independently.*

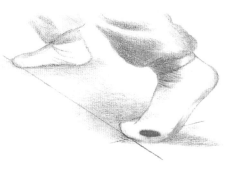

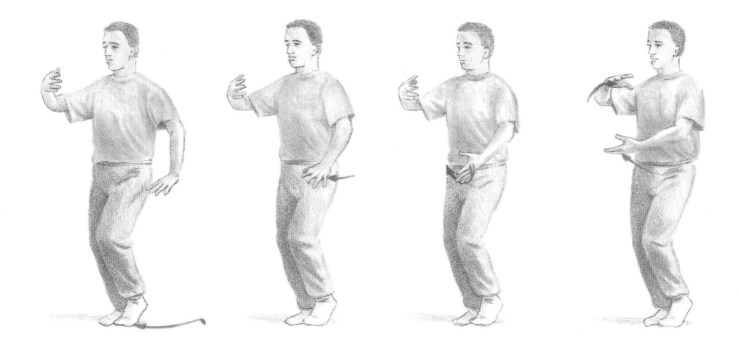

9 Lift your left foot slightly off the ground and move it in a small arc in the direction of your right foot. Bring the ball of your left foot to rest lightly on the ground just beside the instep of your right foot. Your left knee nearly touches your right knee. All your weight is on your right foot.

10 Bring your left hand around in a loose arc at waist level in front of your body, slightly below the level of your navel.

11 As your left hand moves, turn the palm so that it faces upward.

11a Turn your right palm downward so that both palms face each other. It is as if you were now holding a large balloon between your two hands.

11◆ *The centers of both of your palms are in line.*

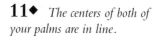

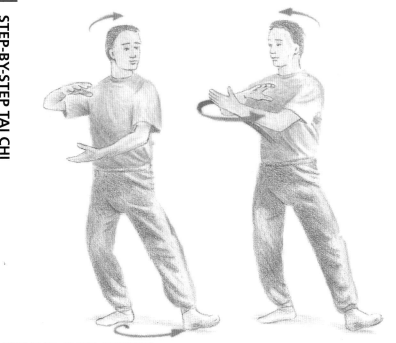
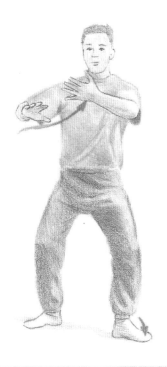
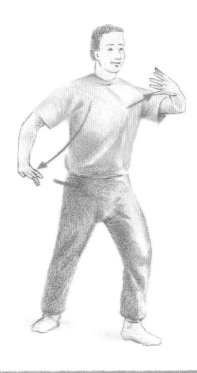

WARD OFF (LEFT)

12 Lift your left foot slightly off the ground. Move it toward the left diagonal. Place your left heel lightly on the ground with the rest of the foot slightly raised. Your weight is on your right foot. Turn your head to the left.

12◆ *The angle between your right heel and left heel is 90 degrees.*

13 Move your left hand inward under your right elbow and then out beneath your forearm. Turn your head to watch your left hand.

13◆ *As you look at your hands, you see the forearms crossed, but not touching.*

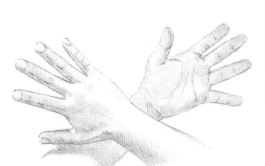

14 Move your left hand toward the left diagonal. Your hips and upper body turn with your arm.

14a Adjust your left forearm so that your palm faces the center of your chest. Imagine you are holding a large balloon between your forearm and your chest. Lower the toes of your left foot back down to the ground and transfer your weight forward. Bring your right hand back and down beside your right hip, the palm facing downward.

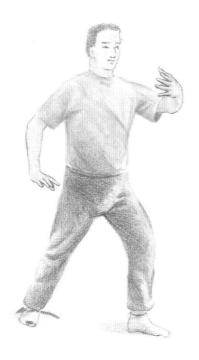

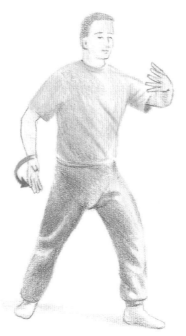

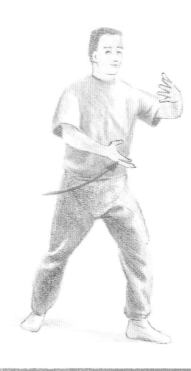

ROLL BACK (LEFT)

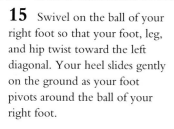

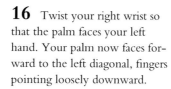

15 Swivel on the ball of your right foot so that your foot, leg, and hip twist toward the left diagonal. Your heel slides gently on the ground as your foot pivots around the ball of your right foot.

16 Twist your right wrist so that the palm faces your left hand. Your palm now faces forward to the left diagonal, fingers pointing loosely downward.

17 Slowly sweep your right hand up. It stops, palm upward, as if it were supporting the imaginary balloon that you hold between your left forearm and your chest.

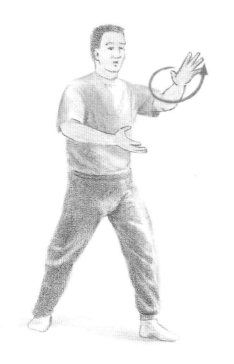
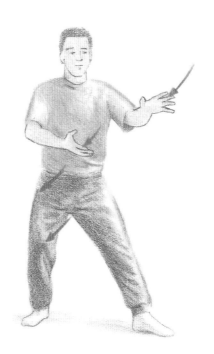
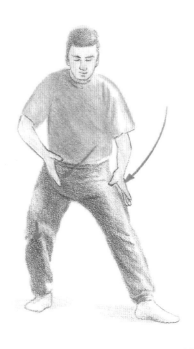

18 Make a small circle with your left hand and reach upward toward the left diagonal.

18◆ *Rotate your left wrist so that your fingers move toward you in the air above your right hand. Continue rotating your wrist so your fingers point downward. Then lift your hand outward and upward toward the left diagonal. The movement ends when you can see the outstretched back of your left hand before you.*

19 Bring your weight down and back on to your right foot. Your right knee bends slightly as the weight transfers to that side of your body.

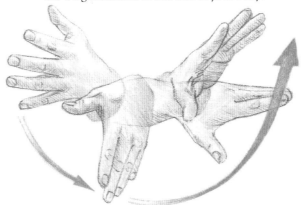

19a Lower both your hands at the same time as if carefully pulling a large object toward your belly. Keep the same distance between your hands as they move. Your right hand stops opposite your lower abdomen. The left hand continues down lower until your arm is nearly straight and your palm is facing downward to your left foot.

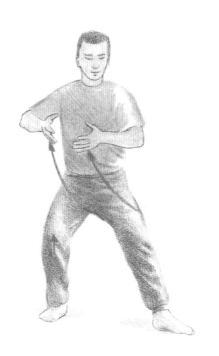

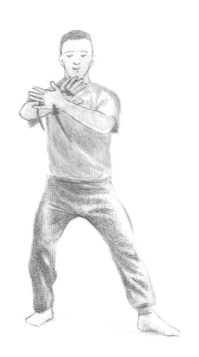

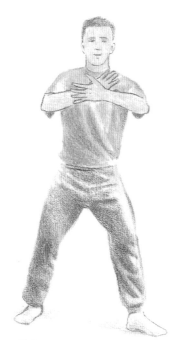

PRESS (LEFT)

20 Keeping the rest of your body still, bend your elbows so that your hands come up toward your chest.

20a Bring the heels of your hands together at the top of the movement, your left hand outermost. As your hands come up, straighten your right knee a little.

21 Use the power in your right leg to start shifting your weight forward on to your left foot. Imagine that the balloon between your arms and chest is starting to expand.

20a◆ *The heels of your hands naturally come together in front of your chest so that your hands are in a crossed position, looking like a butterfly with its wings spread. Both arms should be slightly bent at the elbows. The distance between your hands and the center of your chest should be ample enough to accommodate a balloon in the space.*

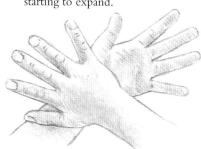

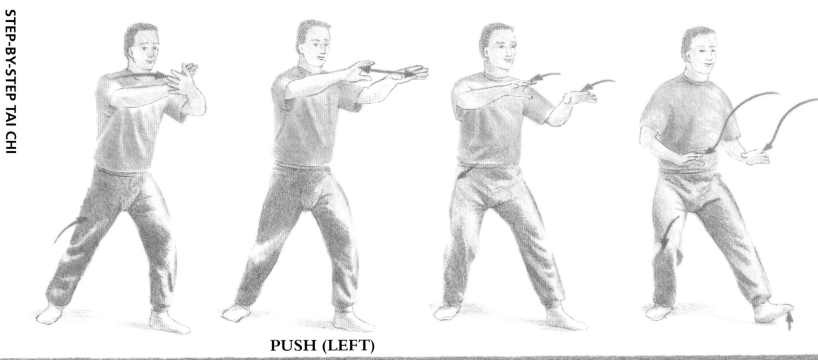

PUSH (LEFT)

21a As you press toward the left diagonal your arms move slightly upward at first and then to chest level as your weight comes forward.

22 Keep your elbows bent. Separate your hands and turn both palms down. Move your two hands away from each other in a horizontal line until they are shoulder-width apart. Your fingers face forward.

23 Your hands remain still. Carefully shift half your weight back on to your right foot. Your torso remains upright as your weight transfers backward.

24 Transfer the rest of your weight on to your right foot. Bend your right knee as you do this. Your torso remains upright but your whole body feels that it is sinking down over the right foot. At the same time, bring both your hands back and down in a diagonal movement toward your waist. The distance between them widens as they come down. Raise your left foot slightly so that only the heel remains on the ground.

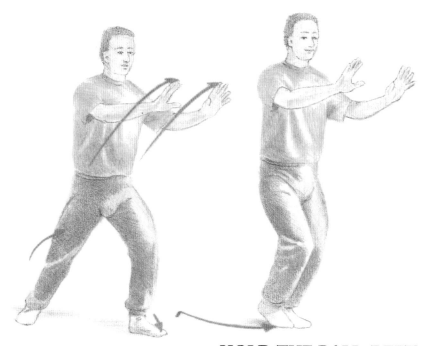 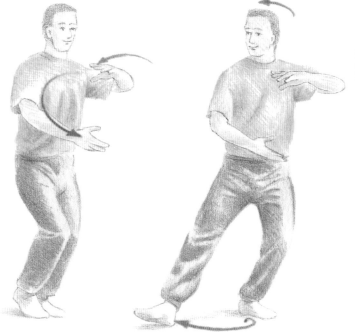

HOLD THE BALL (LEFT)

WARD OFF (RIGHT)

25 Using your right foot, push up and forward. Extend your arms likewise. The distance between your hands narrows to shoulder width. Now your weight has been transferred forward on to your left foot and your lower left leg is roughly at a right-angle to the ground. Your torso should be upright, facing the diagonal. Your hands face forward at 45 degrees, level with your shoulders. Your elbows are gently bent.

26 Keep your arms and body still. All your weight is on your left foot. Now lift your right foot slightly off the ground and move it up beside your left foot. Your right knee nearly touches your left knee. Lightly rest the ball of your right foot on the ground beside the instep of your left foot.

27 Move your left forearm in horizontally toward your chest and turn your left palm downward. Lower your right hand down toward your navel and turn the palm upward. Both palms face each other. It is as if you were now holding a large balloon between your hands.

28 Lift your right foot slightly. Move it away from your left foot toward the right diagonal. Lightly place your right heel on the ground but keep the rest of the foot raised. Your weight is still on your left foot. Turn your head to the right as you move your right foot.

28◆ *The angle between your left heel and right heel is 90 degrees.*

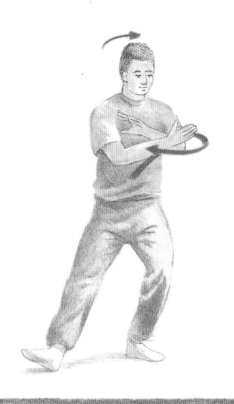

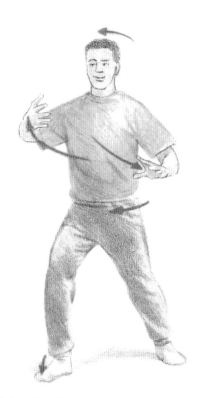

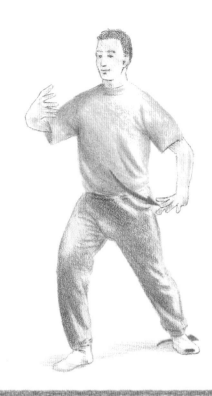

29 Keep your body still. Move your right hand inward under your left elbow and then bring it out beneath your forearm. Your palm faces upward during this movement. When you complete it, you should be able to see your palm facing upward as it extends out from under your left forearm. As you make this movement, turn your head to the left so that you can watch your right hand.

30 Continue the movement of your right hand on toward the right diagonal. Your hips and upper body turn with your arm. As you do this, adjust your forearm so that your right palm faces the center of your chest. Imagine you are holding a large balloon that is starting to expand between your forearm and chest. As your right hand moves, lower the toes of your right foot down to the ground and transfer your weight forward.

31 Swivel on the ball of your left foot so that it twists forward. Bring your left hand back and down beside your left hip, the palm facing downward.

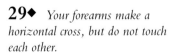

29◆ *Your forearms make a horizontal cross, but do not touch each other.*

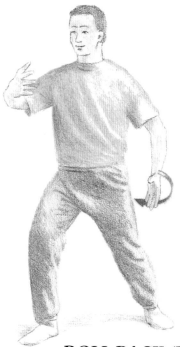

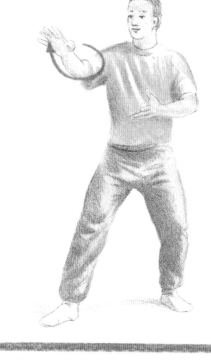

ROLL BACK (RIGHT)

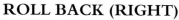

32 Twist your left wrist so that the palm of your left hand faces your right hand. Your palm now faces forward to the right diagonal, fingers pointing loosely downward.

33 Slowly sweep your left hand up. It stops, palm upward, as if it were supporting the imaginary balloon that you hold between your right forearm and your chest.

34 Make a small circle with your right hand and reach upward toward the right diagonal.

34◆ *Rotate your right wrist so that your fingers move toward you in the air above your left hand. Continue rotating your wrist so your fingers point downward. Then lift your hand outward and upward toward the right diagonal. The movement finishes when you can clearly see the outstretched back of your right hand before you.*

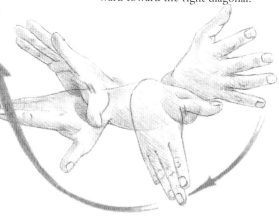

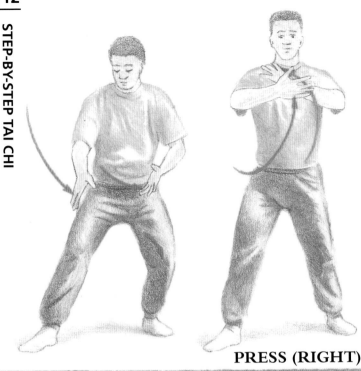

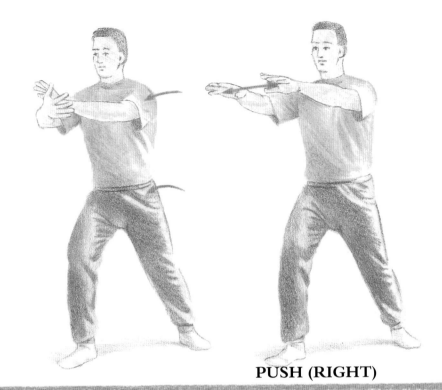

PRESS (RIGHT)

PUSH (RIGHT)

35 Bring your weight down and back on to the left foot. Your left knee bends slightly as the weight transfers to that side. Lower both your hands at the same time as if you were carefully pulling a large object toward your belly. Keep the same distance between your hands as they move. Your left hand stops opposite your lower abdomen. Your right hand continues down lower until your arm is nearly straight and your palm is facing downward to your right foot.

36 Bend your elbows to bring your hands to chest level. The heels of your hands come together, right hand outermost. As your hands rise, straighten your left knee a little.

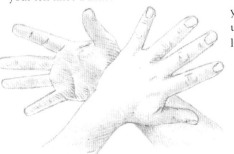

37 Slowly press forward using the power in your left leg to shift your weight forward on to your right foot. Imagine that the balloon between your arms and chest is expanding. This causes your arms to move slightly upward at first and then to chest level as you come forward.

38 Keep your elbows bent. Separate your hands and turn both palms down. Move your hands away from each other in a horizontal line until they are shoulder-width apart. Your fingers face forward.

36◆ *The heels of your hands come together in front of your chest so that your hands are crossed, looking like a butterfly with spread wings. Both arms should be slightly bent. The distance between your hands and chest should be enough to accommodate a balloon.*

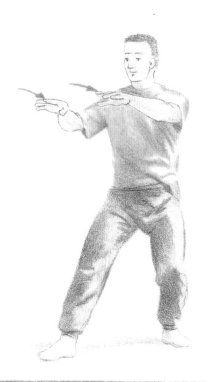

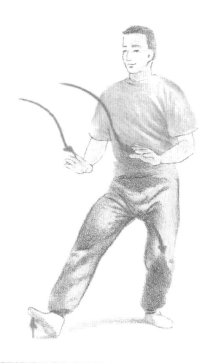

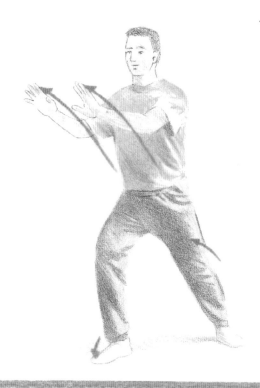

39 Your hands remain still. Carefully shift half your weight back on to your left foot. Your torso remains upright as your weight transfers backward.

40 Transfer the rest of your weight on to your left foot. Bend your left knee as you do this. Your torso remains upright, but your whole body feels that it is sinking down over the left foot. At the same time, bring both your hands back and down in a diagonal movement toward your waist. The distance between them widens as they descend. Raise your right foot slightly so that only the heel remains on the ground.

41 Using your left foot to push forward, steadily push yourself up and forward. Extend your arms so that they move forward and upward. The distance between your hands narrows to shoulder width.

The movement ends when your weight has transferred forward on to your right foot and your lower right leg is roughly at a right-angle to the ground. Your torso should be upright, facing the diagonal. Your hands face forward at a 45-degree angle, level with your shoulders. Your elbows are gently bent.

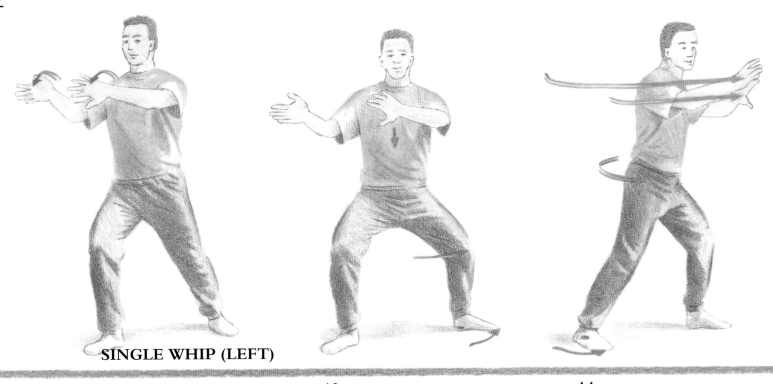

SINGLE WHIP (LEFT)

42 Keep your body still. Turn both your hands to the right, moving only at the wrists, so that your palms turn to face outward.

43 Keep your upper body still, facing the right diagonal. Swivel your left foot on its heel so that the foot opens to point in the direction of the left diagonal. As you do this, bend your knees as if to sit down a little.

44 Swivel your right foot on the heel as far as you can toward the left so that the toes aim at the left diagonal. As you do this, sweep both your arms across in front of your body as if you were moving an object from right to left with your palms. Your hips and upper body move naturally across with the movement of your arms. Your weight shifts across to your left foot. The movement ends when your left wrist is in line with your left knee.

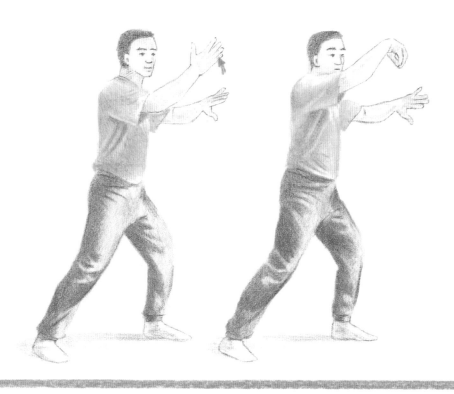

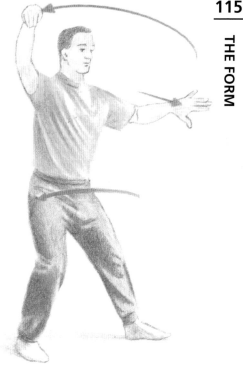

45 Move your right hand in a small horizontal arc in toward your face.

46 Make a "hook" with your right hand.

46◆ *You make the "hook" by gently squeezing the pads of your fingertips against the pad of the tip of your thumb. Turn your wrist so that the fingertips and thumb point downward. Lift the back of your wrist (which is now uppermost) straight up until it becomes the highest raised point of your arm, on a level with your eyes.*

47 Shift your weight from your left foot back over to your right foot. The right knee bends slightly as your weight transfers. Your left knee naturally straightens a little. At the same time lift your "hooked" right hand in a rising arc over to the right, ending up level with the top of your head. As you do this, extend your left hand diagonally downward.

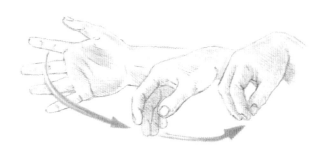

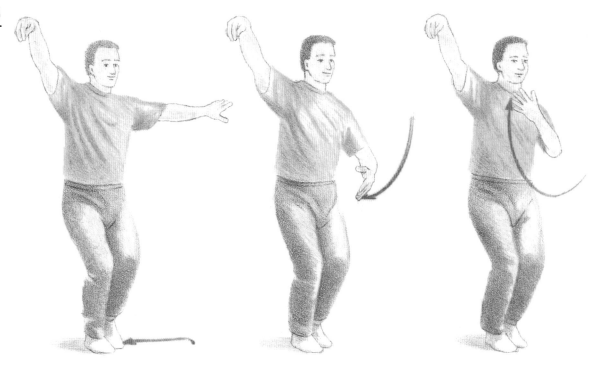
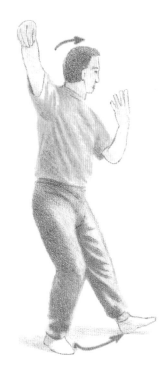

48 Lift your left foot slightly off the ground and move it over toward your right foot. (To do this smoothly, you must be sure that all your weight is balanced firmly on your right foot.) Bring the ball of your left foot to rest lightly on the ground just beside the instep of your right foot. Your left knee nearly touches your right knee.

49 Start to move your left hand downward in a deep arc toward your body.

49a Continue the arc up in front of you so that it finishes with the center of the palm facing the center of your chest. Your fingers are naturally upward.

50 Lift your left foot slightly off the ground. Move it in a wide arc fully around to the left until it points in the direction of the left rear diagonal. Gently rest your left heel on the ground. Your weight still remains firmly on your right foot. Keep the "hook" of your right hand in place. As your foot moves, turn your head to look in the same direction.

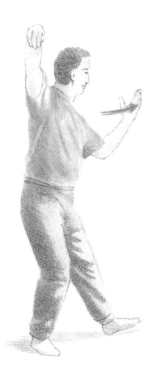

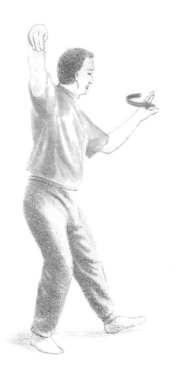

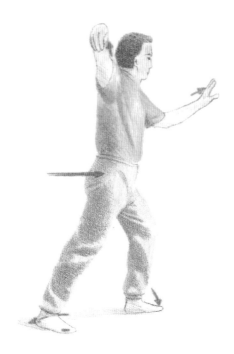

SINGLE WHIP (RIGHT)

51 Move your bent left arm around through the same wide arc as your left foot toward the left rear diagonal until it is in line with your left foot.

52 Gently turn the palm of your left hand to face the left rear diagonal.

53 Transfer your weight forward from your right foot to your left foot. As your weight shifts forward, swivel on the ball of your right foot. Your hips turn with the swivel, twisting the body to face the rear diagonal. Be sure your left knee does not extend over your toes. As you do this, slightly extend your left hand forward away from the "hook" of your right hand and slightly extend your "hook" in the opposite direction.

53◆ *Your left foot points in the direction of the left rear diagonal. Your right foot is turned toward that direction, but not as fully. Note that your right arm, with the right hand still in the "hook" has remained stationary, while the left side of your body has turned away from it toward the left rear diagonal.*

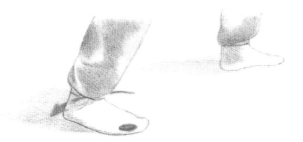

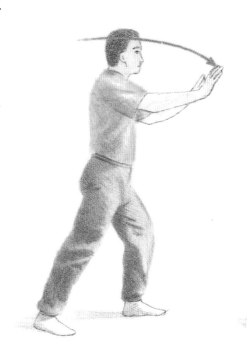

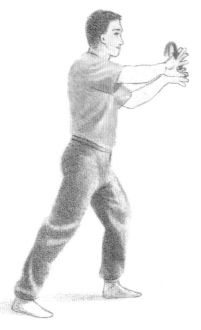

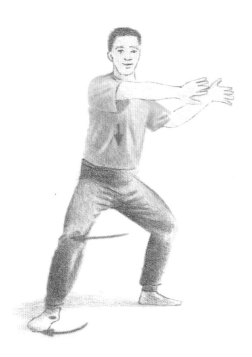

54 Open your right hand. Then, keeping your right elbow in place, gently lower your right forearm to chest level.

55 Turn both your hands to the left, moving only at the wrists, so that the palms of your hands face outward.

56 Keep your upper body still, facing the left diagonal. Swivel your right foot on its heel so that the foot opens to point in the direction of the right diagonal. As you do this, bend your knees as if to sit down a little.

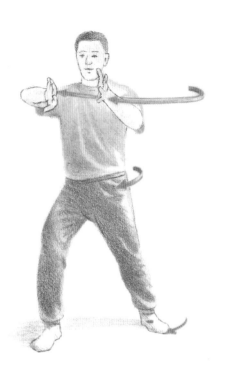

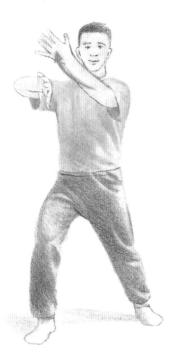

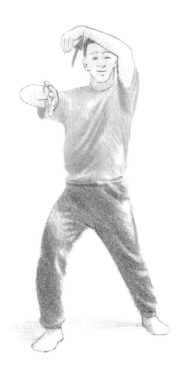

57 Swivel your left foot inward on its heel so that your toes turn toward the right diagonal, but not fully. As you do this, sweep both your arms across in front of your body as if you were moving an object from left to right with your palms. Your hips and upper body move naturally across with the movement of your arms. Your weight shifts across to your right foot. The movement ends when your right wrist is in line with your right knee.

58 Move your left hand in a small horizontal arc in toward your face.

59 Make a "hook" with your left hand as you formerly had done with right hand.

59◆ *The "hook" is made by gently squeezing the pads of your fingertips against the pad of the tip of your thumb. Turn your wrist so that the fingertips and thumb point downward. Lift the back of your wrist (which is now uppermost) straight up until it becomes the highest raised point of your arm, on a level with your eyes.*

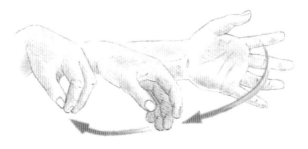

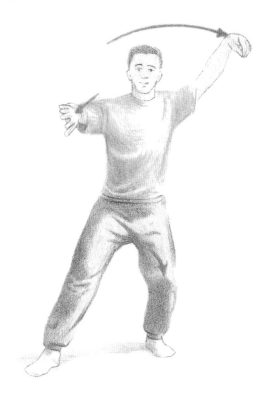

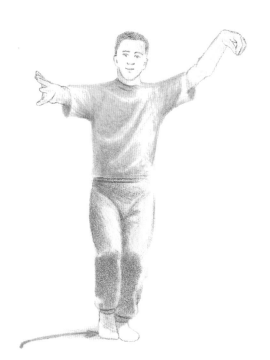

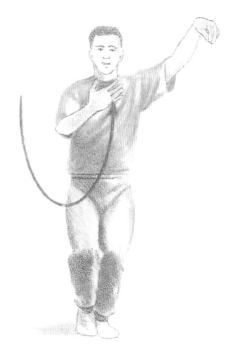

60 Shift your weight from your right foot back over to your left foot. The left knee bends slightly as your weight transfers. Your right knee naturally straightens a little. At the same time lift your left hand "hook" in a rising arc over to the left, ending up level with the top of your head. As you do this, extend your right hand diagonally downward.

61 Lift your right foot slightly off the ground and move it over toward your left foot. (To do this smoothly, you must be sure that all your weight is balanced firmly on your left foot.) Bring the ball of your right foot to rest lightly on the ground just beside the instep of your left foot. Your right knee nearly touches your left knee.

62 Move your right hand in a deep arc down toward your body and then up in front of you so that it finishes with the center of the palm facing the center of your chest. Your fingers are naturally upward.

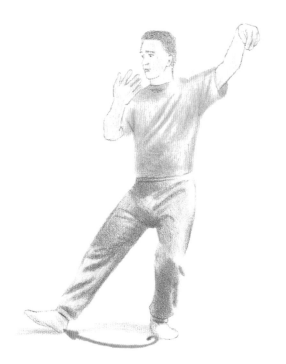

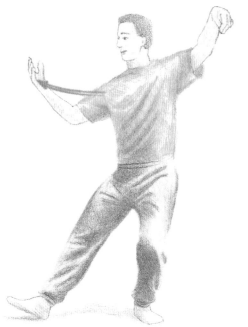

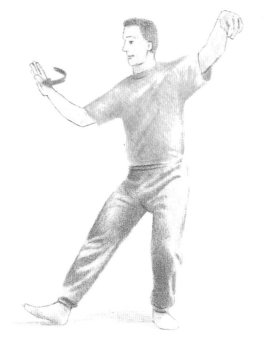

63 Lift your right foot slightly off the ground. Move it in a wide arc around to the right only until it points in to the right side. Gently rest your right heel on the ground. Your weight still remains firmly on your left foot. Keep the raised "hook" of your left hand in place. As your foot moves, turn your head so that it looks in the same direction.

64 Move your bent right arm around to the right side, in line with your right foot.

65 Gently turn the palm of your right hand to face the right side.

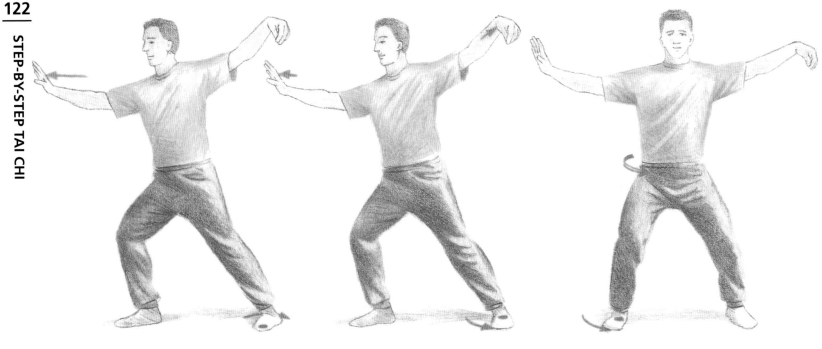

66 Transfer your weight forward from your left foot to your right foot. As your weight shifts forward, swivel on the ball on your left foot. Your hips turn with the swivel, twisting the body to face the right side. Be sure your right knee does not extend over your toes. As you do this, slightly extend your right hand forward away from the "hook" of your left hand and slightly extend your "hook" in the opposite direction.

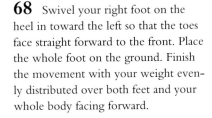

67 Swivel your left foot on the heel a little to the left so that the toes face straight forward to the front. Place the whole foot on the ground.

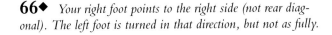

68 Swivel your right foot on the heel in toward the left so that the toes face straight forward to the front. Place the whole foot on the ground. Finish the movement with your weight evenly distributed over both feet and your whole body facing forward.

66◆ *Your right foot points to the right side (not rear diagonal). The left foot is turned in that direction, but not as fully.*

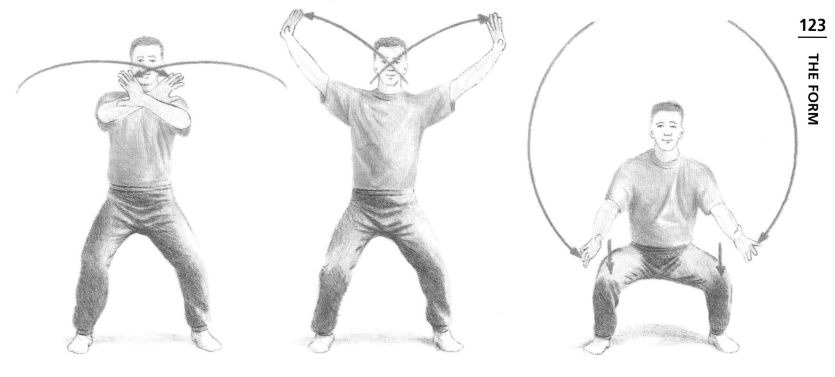

BRING THE TIGER AND RETURN TO THE MOUNTAIN

69 Open your left hand. Cross your arms in front of you and place the inside of your right wrist against the back of your left wrist. The point where both wrists cross each other is level with your neck.

70 From the crossed position, open both of your arms in broad, sweeping arcs, opening fully out to the sides.

70a As your arms start to move downward in the arc, bend your knees as if starting to sit down, keeping your back straight. The palms of your hands should be facing each other.

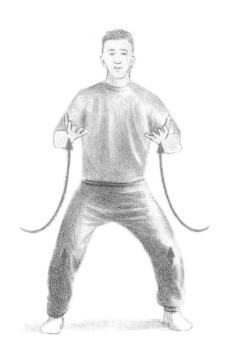

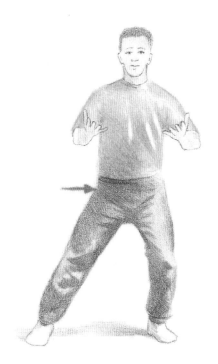

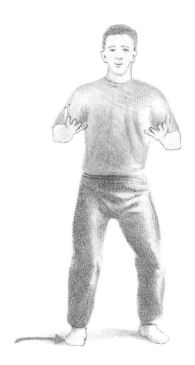

TAI CHI CLOSING

71 Lift both your hands up in front of you as if you were lifting a large, heavy tub. Lift them until they are level with your chest. Keep your shoulders relaxed. As your arms come up, start to stand up.

72 Shift your weight briefly on to your left foot.

72a Lift your right foot slightly off the ground and replace it nearer to your left foot so that your feet are shoulder-width apart. Center your weight directly over both your feet.

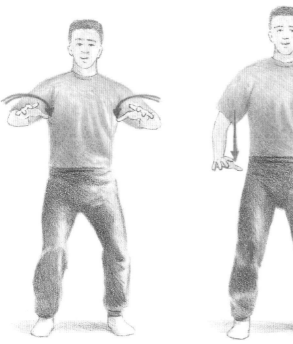
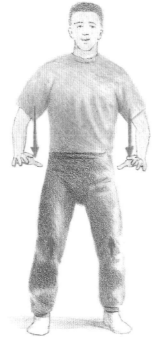
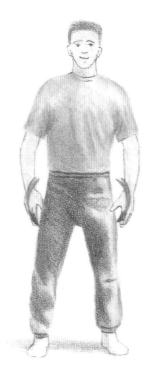

73 Turn both your hands over so that the palms face downward at the level of your chest.

74 Press both your hands slowly downward and in toward your body as if you were pushing a heavy object down into a tub of mud. As your hands slowly descend straighten your knees and stand up. The movement ends when you are standing straight, facing forward. Hands are hip-width apart in front of you, level with your hips, your elbows slightly bent. Your fingers point forward with your palms facing the ground.

75 Let your hands slowly relax down to rest by your sides.

The Tai Chi movement returns to the stillness. Stand quietly for a minute, allowing your internal energies to balance and flow smoothly.

LEARNING THE SMALL CIRCLE FORM

People learn Tai Chi at different rates, even if they go regularly to classes. It is therefore impossible to give a fixed timetable that will meet the different needs and circumstances of all readers. Those who are already familiar with Tai Chi may find that they can pick up the full range of exercises and the Small Circle Form reasonably quickly. From that they will find ways of improving their own Tai Chi practice.

But what about those who are complete beginners? The most important rule is that it is better to go too slow than too fast. The chart on the facing page offers you a step-by-step routine that takes you slowly through half a year. You are free to progress faster if you feel comfortable with that. Conversely, take more time if you feel that is better for you. (You may wish to learn a bit of the Form, go back to allowing more time for the basic Tai Chi exercises for a few weeks, and then pick up the Form where you left off.) Learning and practicing Tai Chi is not a competition: you are not competing against anyone else and please don't treat it as a competition with yourself! The accompanying chart assumes that:

- you have reached an adequate level of suppleness and balance through the preceding exercises (or other similar exercise or previous Tai Chi practice);
- you are prepared to do a little work on your Tai Chi most days, preferably every day;
- you can arrange to spend at least 10 minutes doing basic Tai Chi exercises as a warm up before starting your daily learning;
- you can spend a further 10 minutes studying the instructions and repeating the movements over and over again until you can remember them and perform them without needing to refer to the book.

LEARNING FOR BEGINNERS: STEP-BY-STEP

Week	Movements	Week	Movements
1	Tai Chi Starting: movements 1 – 5	14	Single whip (right): movements 54 – 60
2	Hold the ball (right): movements 6 – 11	15	Single whip (right): movements 61 – 68
3	Ward off (left): movements 12 – 15	16	Bring the tiger and return to the mountain: movements 69 –71
4	Roll back (left): movements 16 – 19		
5	Press (left): movements 20 – 21	17	Tai Chi Closing: movements 72 – 75
6	Push (left): movements 22 – 25	18	Review full sequence of movements 1 – 75
7	Review movements 1 – 25 Check posture advice *(see pp.138, 139)*	19	Repeat form three times; connect movements 1 – 11
		20	Repeat form three times: connect movements 12 – 25
8	Hold the ball (left) and Ward off (right): movements 26 – 31		
		21	Repeat form three times: connect movements 26 – 41
9	Roll back (right) & Press (right): movements 32 – 37		
		22	Repeat form six times: connect movements 42 – 53
10	Push (right): movements 38 – 41	23	Repeat form six times: connect movements 54 – 68
11	Review movements 1 – 41 Check posture advice *(see pp.138, 139)*	24	Repeat form six times: connect movements 69 – 75
		25	Practice whole form with all movements connected, start breathing with the movements *(see p.137)*
12	Single whip (left): movements 42 – 47		
13	Single whip (left): movements 48 – 53	26	Add "Moving the mind" to your form *(see p.140)*

THE MAIN MOVEMENTS

These are the 15 main movements of the Small Circle Form.
Once you have learned the component parts of each of these
movements, you can use this diagram as a general reminder
of the whole sequence of the Form. With practice, it will
become a single, unbroken motion like the opening and
closing of a circle.

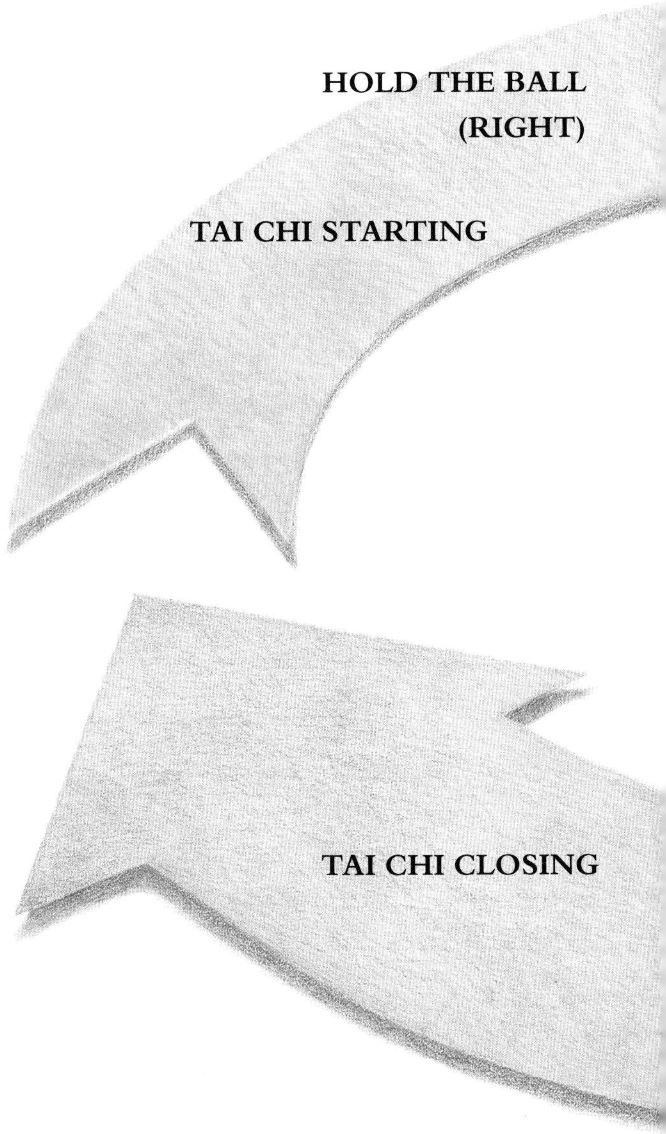

**HOLD THE BALL
(RIGHT)**

TAI CHI STARTING

TAI CHI CLOSING

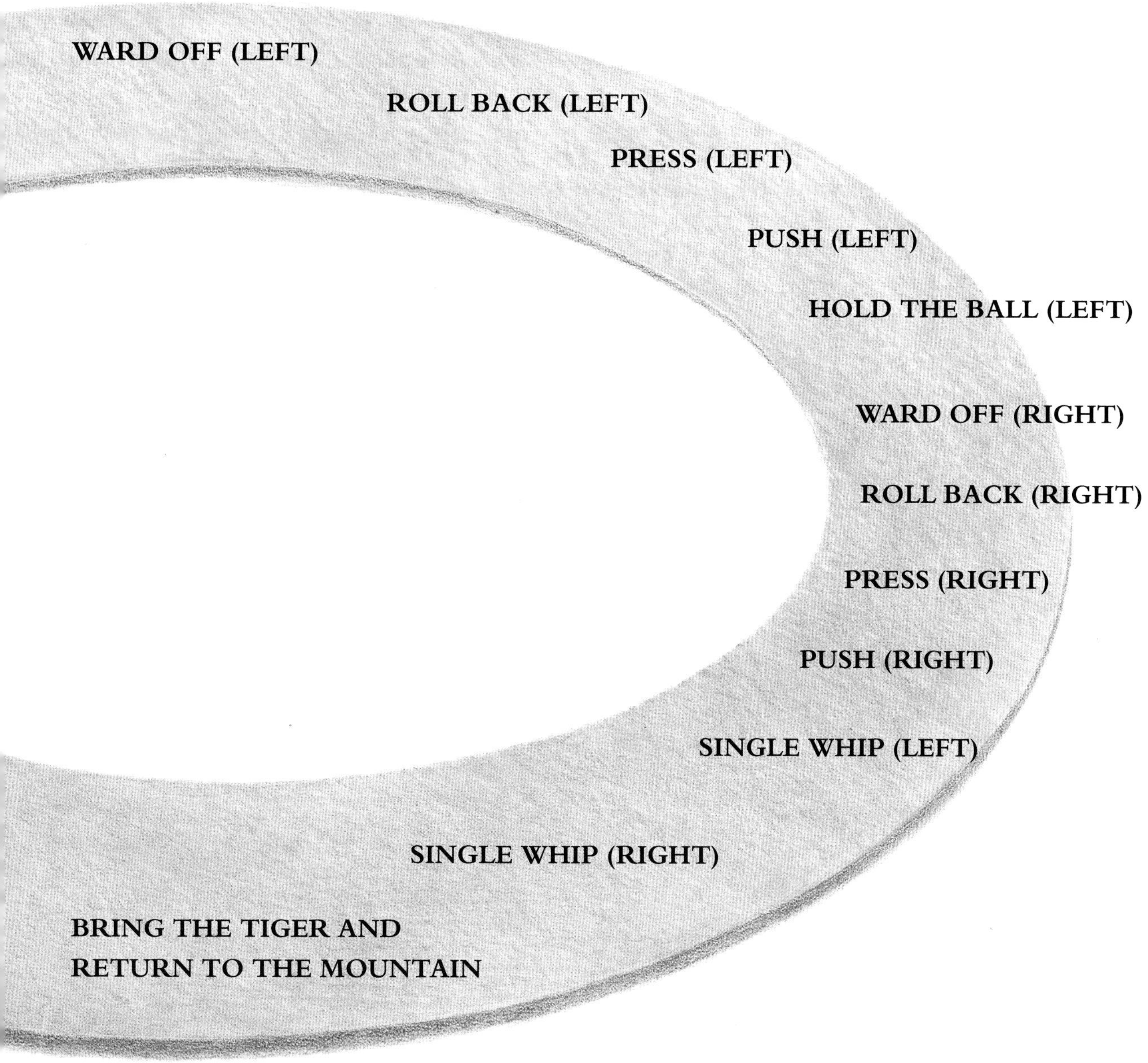

WARD OFF (LEFT)

ROLL BACK (LEFT)

PRESS (LEFT)

PUSH (LEFT)

HOLD THE BALL (LEFT)

WARD OFF (RIGHT)

ROLL BACK (RIGHT)

PRESS (RIGHT)

PUSH (RIGHT)

SINGLE WHIP (LEFT)

SINGLE WHIP (RIGHT)

BRING THE TIGER AND
RETURN TO THE MOUNTAIN

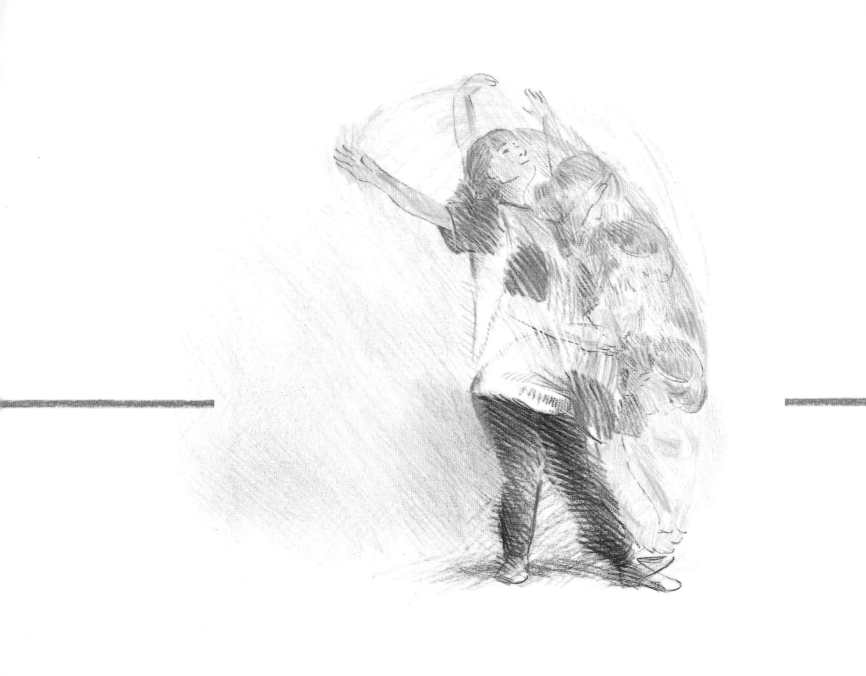

CHAPTER SIX

ONE STROKE OF THE BRUSH

When the great Chinese calligraphers write even the most intricate characters, they soak the brush in the ink, make one stroke of the brush in a single, continuous motion, and the character is completed.

When the great masters perform Tai Chi, they make only one movement. They begin in perfect stillness, move once and are again still. This is what you will learn next on your journey as a Tai Chi student. Each of the tiny individual movements that you have learned in precise detail will become part of a single, flowing movement.

That single motion will not simply be a composite movement of first the arms and then the feet. Your whole body will learn to move as one. As you make progress, your body and your mind will move together.

Having learned the individual movements of the Small Circle Form, the next step is to connect them all together. As you develop in your practice, you will have to pay attention to how the various parts of your body – from your eyes through to your feet – are moving. You will need to learn how to do this in a relaxed way and to harmonize your breathing with your movements. This is essential to ensure complete connection throughout your body.

Although this is the stage at which having a teacher would be of benefit, there are, nevertheless, a number of important points that you can learn on your own. Follow the advice in this chapter and be attentive to what you are actually doing when you practice your Tai Chi. As always, don't be tempted to rush: if you try to accomplish too much too quickly it will be like overwatering a seedling. Just understand one point at a time and, with great care, use it to illuminate what you have learned with such effort so far.

CONNECTING THE MOVEMENTS

Each of the 75 small movements that you have learned in the Small Circle Form is like a numbered dot on a child's puzzle, and you must draw a line through all the dots in order to reveal the hidden image.

You start with number 1 and then move on through all the other numbers at a steady pace without stopping until you have completed number 75. The numbers are like little stops on a railroad. When you were first learning, you stopped at each one. Now you still go to each point, but you pass calmly through it without stopping. The track is the same, but you move along it without pausing.

There is an important difference, however, between mechanical movement on a track and the movement of Tai Chi. The end of each movement in Tai Chi is the beginning of the next. This means that there is a subtle but essential overlap between each and every movement. You do not simply complete number 1 and continue on to number 2. Instead you look carefully at the last few seconds at the end of movement number 1 and the first few seconds at the beginning of movement number 2 and examine how to fuse them together.

You must be sure to complete all of the end of number 1 as well as all of the beginning of number 2, but you will find that you can weld these two together in a perfectly smooth and comfortable join. Without this subtle welding, your Tai Chi will be lifeless. When you have perfected it, the entire sequence will be full, accurate, and intelligent.

The best way to learn this is to take two or three of the individual movements at a time, study their endings and beginnings, and slowly develop the overlapping connections between them. Take a few movements each time you practice over a period of a few weeks. At the end of each week, see if you can connect everything you have worked on during that period.

At this stage people often experience some problems, such as speeding up or starting to cut little bits off the beginnings and endings of movements. Your hands and feet may also move at different speeds, or you may be unstable on your feet and lose your balance a little. The way to avoid these problems is to pay careful attention to making correct, smooth movements in a relaxed way and with your weight "rooted" through your feet.

Sometimes you may find that the length of your steps varies so that your form becomes uneven or lopsided. Try to make steps of equal size and aim to end your form standing in the same place that you began.

This work is mentally absorbing and may be tiring. Just focus your attention on what you are doing for a few minutes at a time, ease off when you are tired, and return to it the next day. In this way you can discover the profound and powerful inner experience of Tai Chi.

STANDING STILL AND RELAXING

Tai Chi movement emerges out of stillness and returns to it. When you practice your Tai Chi movements, to an observer you are moving, but inwardly you are still. These truths are of the utmost importance in your training.

The first stage in your training has been the standing exercise in Chapter Two – Exercise 19 Standing in the Wu Chi Position (*see p.42*). This is the first, fundamental position of the Zhang Zhuang system of Chi Kung. Zhan Zhuang, pronounced "Jan Jong" in Chinese, literally means "Standing Like a Tree".

When you stand still in this position, with your body correctly aligned between the ground and the sky, you are drawing energy (chi) from the two great forces of heaven and earth. The first known reference to this profound system of internal exercise dates back to the most influential book ever written in the history of world medicine, *The Yellow Emperor's Classic of Internal Medicine* (Huang Ti Nei Ching), which is thought to have been written some 4000 years ago. This exercise, and its importance, are fully explained in *The Way of Energy*, published by Gaia Books.

Once you have connected the movements of the Small Circle Form into a single, flowing sequence, you should make a serious effort to increase the internal development of your energy by standing in the Wu Chi position for between two and nine minutes before beginning your form.

Use the time you spend standing to relax your whole body. Begin with the skin and muscles around your eyes; mentally check for tension and encourage full relaxation there. Move down to the angles of your jaw; make sure you are not clenching your teeth. Then let the sense of relaxation travel down the sides of your neck. Take your mind to your right shoulder; let it sink down; feel your right hand hanging heavily by your side. Then go over to your left shoulder and let it sink down as well. On your next outbreath, exhale fully so that your chest sinks inward. Then imagine that a soothing stream of clear water is washing down your back, carrying any obstructions away with it. Feel the downward movement pass through your buttocks; relax the muscles. You will feel as if more and more of your weight is sinking to the soles of your feet.

Then take your mind to the very top of your head, to a point in line with the tips of your ears. Imagine that your head is suspended from a fine golden thread, your body hanging gently below. You are poised between heaven and earth.

Once you have completed this essential practice, smoothly begin your form. When you complete your form, stand still for a further minute or two.

BREATHING

Breathing and movement go together in Tai Chi. As you develop, your movement will become an expression of your breath. There are two stages in developing Tai Chi breathing. The first stage is to focus your breathing on the point known in Chinese as the Tan Tien, which is approximately 2 inches (5cm) below your navel. Practice this abdominal breathing by folding your hands over your abdomen below the navel. As you breathe in, imagine that the air is going deep inside you and feel your belly filling up under your hands. As you breathe out, press in slightly with your hands to help your belly move inward.

Allow these movements to happen calmly. Just relax – close your eyes if that helps at first – and feel the expanding and then slight contracting movements of your belly. You may find that it helps to concentrate more on your outbreath: your inbreath will take care of itself.

Practice this while standing still for a couple of minutes each day. When you have developed your form to the point where it is reasonably smooth, you can work with your breath while moving. The underlying principles are simple. Try following the general principles outlined in the chart opposite.

If you find the rate of breathing is too slow at some points, you can try adding a little in-and-out breath wherever you need it between the movements. If you find it difficult to add in the breathing in this way at this stage, just go back to what you were doing before. It is more important to be smooth and relaxed than to worry about your breathing.

BREATHING AND MOVEMENT

Tai Chi Starting	As you begin and your arms come up, breathe in. As your arms press down, breathe out.
Hold the Ball	As your arm comes up and you swivel, breathe in. As you step up and hold the ball, breathe out.
Ward Off	As you step to the diagonal, breathe in. As you move your arm outward and transfer your weight forward, breathe out.
Roll Back	As you bring your hand up, breathe in. As you bring your hands back down, breathe out.
Press On	As you bring your hands up together, breathe in. As you press forward, breathe out.
Push	As your hands separate and come back down, breathe in. As you push up, breathe out.
Single Whip	As you sit down, breathe in. As you sweep across, breathe out. As you make the hook and scoop up, breathe in. As you step out and push forward, breathe out.
Bring Tiger & Return to the Mountain	As you face forward and cross your wrists, breathe in. As you scoop down, breathe out. As you rise up, breathe in.
Tai Chi Closing	As you turn your hands over, press down and stand up, breathe out.

POSTURE AND GESTURE

As you practice the flowing movement of the Form, pay attention to each of the following elements of your body. Select one to practice each day and check to see if you need to make any correction to your posture or movement.

Your eyes
Your eyes are alert, paying attention to the movement of your hands, using your full field of vision.

Your nose
Breathe quietly in and out through your nostrils, not through your mouth.

Your head
Your head is held upright by a fine golden thread rising from the crown.

Your chin
Allow the chin to rest in its natural, slightly downward position.

Your hips
Visualise 70 percent of your body weight sinking below your hips; 30 percent rides above, like a rider on a horse.

Your knees
Do not bend your knees so far that they extend forward over your toes.

Your hands
Because the Zhan Zhuang system of Chi Kung is embedded deep inside the Small Circle Form, when your hands are open, your fingers should always be gently apart as if there were tiny balls resting in between them.

Your mouth
Your teeth and lips are gently closed with the tip of the tongue resting naturally behind your upper teeth.

Your shoulders
Relaxation of your shoulders is essential. They have a tendency to rise up unnoticed, drawing energy upward in the body, causing tension and headaches. Devote care to relaxing them throughout your form.

Your arms
Your elbows and wrists should be sufficiently relaxed so that your arm is never stiffly extended with the joints locked.

Your back
Your lower back feels as if it is sinking downward. To avoid sticking your backside out, tuck the bottom of your spine slightly in.

YOUR MIND AND ENERGY

Tai Chi is an exercise of the mind. Your mind directs your energy. The movement of your energy is the movement of Tai Chi.

A tranquil mind and smooth, flowing energy will develop as you go further in your Tai Chi practice. They are the basis of all health in Chinese medicine and the foundation of power in the martial arts. You can enhance these qualities with regular practice.

MOVING THE MIND

Imagine that you are moving first in a tank of water, later in a tank of oil. As you practice your form, use your mind to create the effects of the liquid through which your entire body is moving. No action can be performed quickly. All movements are heavy. As your arm moves forward, it feels the resistance of the liquid. At the same time, the liquid flows in behind it to support it. Feel the movements of the liquid as you turn and rock forward and backward. Later, you may come to feel as if the liquid is inside you and that your body moves with the wave-like flow of the liquid and not with the use of muscle.

CHI KUNG IN YOUR TAI CHI

Go back to the very beginning of your study of the Small Circle Form. Begin with Standing in the Wu Chi Position for several minutes. Then move slowly through each of the 75 little movements of the Form. At the end of each one, hold your position for 10 seconds without moving. This is extremely powerful. You should attempt it only after a year of regular practice of your form. Try doing it once a week. If you feel any unpleasant symptoms, ease off and go back to your normal practice next day.

A second approach is first to stand in the Wu Chi position for several minutes and then to do the Small Circle Form three times in succession, pausing only very briefly between each repetition of the Form. First, go through the Form simply to refresh your memory. Next, do it paying particular attention to your positions and technique. Finally, just let yourself flow through the Form.

When you do the Form after standing in the Wu Chi position, try to sustain the sense of rooting through your feet, the slight sense of upward suspension at the top of your head, and relaxation throughout your entire body. Feel the same sense of inner stillness that you had when standing as you move through the Form.

DEVELOPING YOUR PRACTICE

If you have got this far in your practice, you may wonder what to do next. If you can find a good instructor, you will benefit enormously. You will bring the benefits of everything you have learned and your instructor will help you to build on that foundation. But if you are alone and without the possibility of further instruction, you can refine your Tai Chi and your energy by the constant and regular attention that you devote to your practice. Follow the advice in this book. In the words of one of the greatest books of wisdom in the East: "Work with diligence and care and the light in you will grow."

RESOURCES

Instruction

The New York Open Center, 83 Spring St. New York, NY (212-219-2527)

T'ai Chi Studio, 81 Spring St. New York, NY (212-226-6664)

T'ai Chi Chuan Center, 125 West 43rd St. New York, NY (212-221-6110)

The School of T'ai Chi Chuan, 5 East 17th St. New York, NY (212-929-1981)

The School of T'ai Chi Chuan offers classes at many locations throughout the United States. In your area, contact:

Amherst, MA (413-549-4499)	Atlanta, GA (404-843-9531)	Baltimore, MD (301-962-1308)
Chicago, IL (312-989-0069)	Gainesville, FL (904-371-7234)	Detroit, MI (313-665-1188)
Jacksonville, FL (904-285-4433)	Ludlow, VT (802-228-4506)	Montclair, NJ (201-783-5221)
Los Angeles, CA (310-306-2864)	Portland, OR (503-246-4131)	Spokane, WA (509-747-6401)
Washington, D.C. (703-845-0083)	New York City (212-929-1981)	

Author's details

Details of other instructional materials are available from: The Lam Association, 1 Hercules Road, London. SE1 7DP Telephone/Fax +44 20 7261 9049; Mobile +44 7831 802 598

PUBLISHER'S ACKNOWLEDGMENTS

The publishers would like to express their thanks to all those people who have helped to make this book. Special thanks go to Susan Walby, Suzy Boston, Lucy Guenot, Lesley Gilbert, Master Look, Cristina Masip, Fiona Trent, and all the models Master Lam has mentioned on page 5, particularly Sarah Vicary for her hard work and patience during the photo shoot for the front cover.

FURTHER READING

BOOKS

Jou, Tsung Hwa, *The Tao of Tai-Chi Chuan*, Tai Chi Foundation, Warwick, New York, 1981

Lam, Kam Chuen, *The Way of Energy*, Simon & Schuster, New York, 1991

Jou, Taung H., *The Tao of Tai-Chi Chuan: Way to Rejuvenation*, Tuttle, Charles M., Company, 1981

Reid, Howard, *The Way of Harmony*, Simon & Schuster, New York, 1989

Lee, Martin and Emily, *Ride the Tiger to the Mountain: Tai Chi for Health*, Addison-Wesley Publishing Co., Massachusetts, 1989

Lo, Pang Jeng, *The Essence of T'ai Chi Ch'uan*, North Atlantic Books, Berkeley, California, 1985

Liang, T.T., *T'ai Chi Ch'uan for Health and Self-Defense: Philosophy and Practice*, Random House, New York, 1977

MAGAZINES

Smalheiser, Marvin (ed.), "T'ai Chi", Wayfarer Publications, Los Angeles